THE FRIENDS AND FAMILY GUIDE TO THE OPIOID OVERDOSE EPIDEMIC

The Friends and Family Guide

to the Opioid Overdose Epidemic

Including
How to Recognize and Treat
an Overdose

PETER CANNING

Johns Hopkins University Press
Baltimore

© 2025 Peter Canning
All rights reserved. Published 2025
Printed in the United States of America on acid-free paper
9 8 7 6 5 4 3 2 1

Johns Hopkins University Press
2715 North Charles Street
Baltimore, Maryland 21218
www.press.jhu.edu

Library of Congress Cataloging-in-Publication Data is available.

ISBN 978-1-4214-5284-5 (paperback)
ISBN 978-1-4214-5285-2 (ebook)

A catalog record for this book is available from the British Library.

Special discounts are available for bulk purchases of this book.
For more information, please contact Special Sales at specialsales@jh.edu.

EU GPSR Authorized Representative
LOGOS EUROPE, 9 rue Nicolas Poussin, 17000, La Rochelle, France
E-mail: Contact@logoseurope.eu

*To the men and women of the Connecticut
Harm Reduction Alliance, and all those
in harm reduction, standing in the gap.*

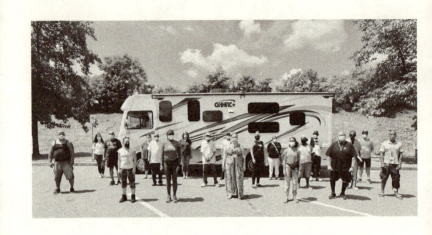

Into whatsoever house I enter, I will enter
to help the sick.
—Hippocratic Oath

CONTENTS

Author's Note   xiii

Introduction   1

PART ONE   How to Recognize and Treat Overdose

1. Overdose: Who Is at Risk   17

   Bread   31

2. How to Recognize Overdose   32

   Wrestler   42

3. Naloxone   45

   Mother   67

4. 911 and Beyond   70

   Mate   81

PART TWO   Understanding the Crisis

5. Fentanyl: The Present Danger   87

   Mascot   113

6. Why People Use Drugs and the Science of Addiction   114

   Emerald City   122

7. Treatment and Recovery   125

   Pink Froth   137

8 **Harm Reduction: Keeping People Alive** 139

A Ravine in Winter 148

9 **The Harms of Stigma** 150

A Confrontation 160

10 **Ending the War on People/Hope for the Future** 163

A Diamond 178

Epilogue: My Brother's Keeper 180

Change 185

PART THREE Action

Key Points: 10 Lessons from This Book 191

Action Plan: A Seven-Point Agenda to Address the Crisis 193

Acknowledgments 197
Glossary 201
A Note on Sources 215
About the Author 249
Illustration Credits 251
Index 253

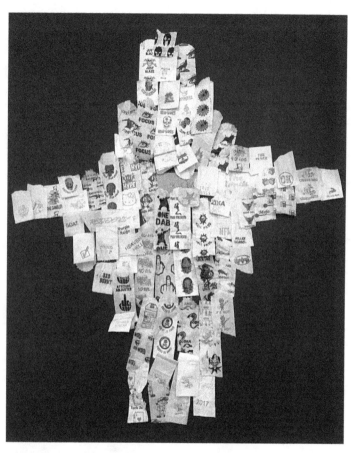

"Forsaken"

AUTHOR'S NOTE

This book is intended for the general public to educate citizens about the opioid epidemic in an accessible, easy-to-read format. It is not a scholarly treatise, but I have included a detailed section on many of the sources I used that readers can refer to should they wish to explore further. Additional photos and videos can be viewed at https://www.petercanning.org/disc.htm.

I have done my best to avoid judgmental stigmatizing language, which can be harmful, as I explain in chapter 9. *Substance use* is the preferred term to *substance abuse*. While "people who use drugs" is preferred to "user," writing "person who uses drugs" in every instance clutters the writing and does not always reflect talk in real life.

In between chapters, I have included short street scenes to remind us that while science and data can tell us much about the grand view of the epidemic, the crisis is striking down individuals. The stories are true. Some details have been changed to protect confidentiality.

THE FRIENDS AND FAMILY GUIDE
TO THE OPIOID OVERDOSE EPIDEMIC

Introduction

My name is Peter Canning. I am a 911 paramedic who has responded to drug overdoses for more than 30 years. I have witnessed the trajectory of the opioid epidemic that cost a record 107,941 Americans their lives in 2022. They died not because more people are using street drugs today but because it has never been more dangerous to use these drugs. Fentanyl, a synthetic opioid 50 times stronger than heroin, has poisoned the illicit drug supply. Fentanyl is too concentrated for drug dealers to properly mix. Two percent fentanyl in one counterfeit (fake) Percocet or in a 0.1 gram bag of powder, which goes for as little as $2, is considered a potentially lethal dose. Without the ability to gauge what percentage of fentanyl is in the purchased pill or powder, anyone using a drug containing fentanyl, from novice pill popper to experienced intravenous drug user, is at risk for overdose and death. In the age of fentanyl, the only way to prevent death is to never use alone and always have naloxone, the opioid antidote, available for administration if overdose occurs. This is the hard truth.

In 2015, in my role as an emergency medical services (EMS) coordinator, I read the following excerpt from another paramedic's patient care report:

> *Upon arrival found a 24 Y/O female unresponsive lying on the floor of her bedroom with her father performing CPR on her. He states that he last saw her alive an hour ago and then found her on the floor unconscious before calling 911. He states she has a history of heroin use, and there is a used needle on the ground next to her. She is unresponsive, with no palpable pulse, and she is apneic.*

A father performing CPR on his daughter is tragic, but grimmer was my realization that such scenes had become commonplace. I had read similar run forms, and as a working paramedic, I had been on these calls.

The sheer number of overdoses we were responding to—driven by fentanyl and increasing with each passing year—had grown impossible to ignore. In 1995, when I started full-time work as a 911 paramedic in Hartford, Connecticut, there were 12,779 fatal overdoses in the country. By 2015, the number was 52,404, a fourfold increase. In Connecticut alone the number of overdose fatalities doubled in just three years between 2012 and 2015. As the 1970s Stephen Stills anthem "For What It's Worth" demanded, it was time to stop and look around.

I once believed that people who used drugs had character flaws and were to blame for their own actions and fates, but

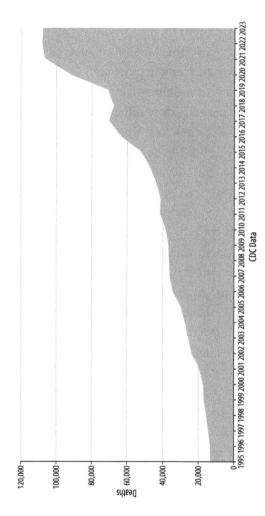

The span of the epidemic: US annual overdose deaths, 1995–2023. Overdose fatalities per year in the United States rose from 12,779 in 1995 when I started as a paramedic in Hartford to 107,543 in 2023.

as the overdoses mounted with no end in sight, I began to wonder if there were larger forces at fault.

I started asking questions. I talked to doctors, substance use experts, and law enforcement personnel. I read books, reports, and research articles in medical journals. Only when I began asking my patients, "How did you start using opioids in the first place?" and then listening to their answers did I begin to truly understand the causes of the epidemic. These were regular people, once no different from you or me. Their heart-wrenching stories of the perilous and unintended paths their lives took changed the way I felt about drug use, addiction, mental health, and the War on Drugs.

Three patients particularly stood out.

A thin girl with long unwashed black hair slumped over the wheel of her crashed car. Tattoos of long-stemmed roses on her arms covered the marks made by needles like the one I found on the floorboard, next to an empty heroin bag branded "Sweet Dreams." After I revived her with naloxone, she expressed dismay at the hurt her father would feel when he heard she had relapsed again. She looked familiar to me, and when she told me she had broken her back cheerleading a few years before, I remembered her. We transported her to the hospital, and I assured her dad, who rode with us, that she would be okay. She told me she had had surgery and was out of school for months. She took more pills than she should have because the pills helped her forget the pain and all she was missing. After escalating her prescription several times, her doctor finally cut her off, telling her she should no longer have a need for painkillers. Feeling sick from withdrawal, she bought pills from a friend at school, but they were expensive. Soon, the same guy who had sold her the pills sold her heroin, which was much cheaper and stronger. She had been to rehab twice for her addiction and was no doubt headed for a third visit. I saw her father again when he arrived in the emergency department (ED). Instead of yelling at her, he embraced her as they both fought back tears. "We'll beat this," he told her. "We'll beat this."

Acquaintances picked up the young man when he was released from jail following 15 days for failure to appear on a trespassing warrant. They gave him a $4 bag of heroin, which he snorted. He had not used opioids in three months, having finally found the strength to battle the withdrawals of the drugs that had destroyed his life. With his tolerance gone, the one bag that might have produced a pleasant, euphoric high when he had been using regularly now stopped his breathing. His acquaintances drove to the entrance of an old hospital that no longer had an ED, pushed him out the car door onto the pavement, and left him. A security guard found him and called 911, and the first responders resuscitated him with naloxone. "After all I've been through, to almost die like this," he said to us on the way to the hospital. "What a scumbag I am. I was supposed to take my daughter trick-or-treating tonight." We noticed a circular scar on his chest. He told us he had been shot in Iraq following an ambush where his Humvee hit an improvised explosive device. He had enlisted in the army the day after 9/11 and came home with a Purple Heart and an addiction to pain pills. He could not hold a job. His wife divorced him, taking custody of his child. When he was not staying on other people's couches, he lived in a tent in the woods. At the hospital, after the nurse shook her head when I said I was bringing her an OD (an overdose patient), I told her his story, knowing her husband had also fought in Iraq. With that knowledge, she and others in the ED who heard his story made a point of going into his room and thanking him for his service. It took a story for them to overcome a stereotype. The more individual stories I heard, the more I came to understand that everyone had a story and was deserving of empathy.

A new face on Park Street, a woman held up a cardboard sign that read "Homeless and Hungry." She looked drug-sick. She was pale and jittery. I could see the track marks on her arms. My partner and I gave her an apple and some change we had in our pockets. We saw her later that day, and she thanked us. When I saw her again later that week, I asked her how she started using opioids. She said when she was young her mother gave her up for heroin, leaving her to be raised by her grandmother. She said she had always wanted to try heroin so she could see what it was about the drug that would make her mother love it more than her own daughter. When the woman tried it, she said she finally understood her mother. That is how powerful the drug is. And now here she was in her mid-thirties, living the same life her mother had, an unhoused sex worker.

These three and others like them put personal faces on the epidemic for me. None of them woke up and decided to become addicted to opioids. Over and over I heard the phrase, "I used to be a normal person once." Their journeys often started with a car accident, a sports injury, a fall off a ladder, or a cancer surgery. For others, it was simple experimentation. Whether it was a trusted doctor giving them an opioid prescription for six months and then upping their doses when they built a tolerance or simply a friend giving them pills to help them forget physical or emotional pain, the unlucky ones were ensnared on paths they could not have foreseen. Eventually cut off from their prescriptions or supply and tormented by the pangs of withdrawal, many sought relief where they could. Ingesting pills led to crushing them and snorting the powder, and then often to the more dangerous method of injecting. Prescription pills like oxycodone led to the cheaper, stronger, and more readily available heroin. Instead of finding empathy or help from the world they knew, they were driven into the shadows, stigmatized as junkies, addicts, and criminals. Many lost their jobs, their homes, their families, and their friends. Some lost their lives. Most who died died alone. Some died under bridges and behind dumpsters, others in their childhood bedrooms. Paramedics like me stood over their lifeless bodies, running six-second strips of asystole (flatline) on our cardiac monitors before covering the bodies with white sheets.

As bad as conditions were in 2015, they were about to get much worse. Fentanyl, a synthetic opioid, visibly indistinguishable from powdered white heroin, had begun to poison the drug supply. Previously, fentanyl had been used on rare occasions as an adulterant to heroin to increase a batch's strength. Along much of the East Coast, where the predominant form of heroin was powder rather than the unrefined black tar heroin used more commonly west of the Mississippi, fentanyl began to replace heroin. The change was driven not by user demand but by economics. Fentanyl didn't have to be grown; it could be manufactured, thus ensuring an unlimited supply. And because fentanyl is 50 times stronger than heroin by weight, it was easier to smuggle into the country. A kilogram of pure fentanyl is equivalent in potency and profit to 50 kilos of heroin. In Connecticut in 2012, there were 14 overdose deaths attributable to fentanyl. By 2021, fentanyl would kill 1,312 people that year alone, representing 86 percent of all overdose deaths.

My experiences and my patients' stories propelled me to write *Killing Season: A Paramedic's Dispatches from the Front Lines of the Opioid Epidemic*, which was published in April 2021.

With the death toll still rising and with so much misinformation about the epidemic being propagated on the news, I was encouraged to write a second book to specifically offer a guidebook for Americans whose families and friends have been affected by the crisis. Who is at risk for addiction? How do you recognize an overdose? How do you obtain and use the lifesaving drug naloxone, also known as Narcan? What are the treatment options for someone with substance use disorder? How does stigma affect our view of people who use drugs? What is harm reduction? And what can we do as a society to end this crisis? This is the same information I now regularly share on emergency scenes.

After being resuscitated, a 23-year-old man told me of his homelessness and of his struggle with opioids that began with a skiing injury. He said the drugs made him feel whole in a way he had never felt before, and they helped him escape his shame of being sexually abused at the hands of a teacher in junior high school. On the way to the hospital, I told him not to give up on rehab, which he had already been to twice before slipping up again. If he was going to use opioids, I told him where he could get clean needles and how to obtain naloxone. And make certain to never use alone, I said. This was not advice he was accustomed to hearing from anyone, much less someone in a uniform. "Why do you care about me?" he asked. I told him I used to not treat overdose patients particularly well, but I knew better now. His addiction was not a character flaw but a medical disease. I explained to him how childhood trauma made some people particularly vulnerable. "You should talk to my parents," he said. "They think I'm a loser."

This book is written for that young man, his parents, and others like them. It is written for all the family members and friends who have witnessed drug use affect the lives of their loved ones and who now want accurate information to better understand the epidemic so they can take action to help save lives. The book is also written for people like I used to be, who thought the threat of arrest should be enough to stop people from using drugs and who judged people's character without knowing the history of the epidemic, the science of addiction, or the stories behind individuals' descents into drug use. Finally, it is written for our policymakers to help them better understand what is happening on the streets and urge them to abandon the usual political "Lock them up!" talking points and instead to embrace evidence-based solutions.

This book is divided into three sections. Part One explains how to recognize and treat overdose. Part Two is a guide to the opioid crisis. The Conclusion includes key points, an action plan, and a glossary.

Here is a brief summary of what you will learn in each chapter:

PART ONE: HOW TO RECOGNIZE AND TREAT OVERDOSE

Chapter 1: Overdose: Who Is at Risk

According to the National Center for Drug Abuse Statistics, close to 60 million Americans use illegal drugs or misused prescription pills annually. An estimated 27 million struggle with substance use disorder. I discuss the risk factors that can lead to drug use, addiction, overdose, and death.

Chapter 2: How to Recognize Overdose

From prescription pills like Percocet and oxycodone to illicit street drugs like heroin and fentanyl, opioids bring pleasure and pain relief in small doses but can easily cause unconsciousness, depressed breathing, and death if too much is taken. I explain how opioids affect the brain and body, how to recognize an overdose, and what to do when confronted with one.

Chapter 3: Naloxone

Naloxone is an opioid antidote that can be easily administered by anyone during an emergency. I explain how naloxone works, where to obtain it, and how to administer it. I also address various myths about naloxone, including claims that naloxone encourages drug use.

Chapter 4: 911 and Beyond

Whenever naloxone has been administered, 911 should always be activated. I explain what to expect when you call 911 to report an overdose, the actions emergency medical services will take, and how opioid overdose patients are cared for at the hospital once they are brought in by ambulance.

PART TWO: UNDERSTANDING THE CRISIS

Chapter 5: Fentanyl: The Present Danger

Fentanyl represents the third and deadliest wave of the opioid crisis. I discuss the dangers of fentanyl, heroin, and other opioids, as well as the newer threats of fake pills containing fentanyl, fentanyl-contaminated cocaine, and the horse tranquilizer xylazine. I also address many of the sensational myths surrounding fentanyl (and the negative effects of those myths), including first responders becoming sick from fentanyl "exposure," fentanyl-contaminated marijuana, and reports of drug dealers targeting children with "rainbow fentanyl."

Chapter 6: Why People Use Drugs and the Science of Addiction

People use drugs because drugs work for whatever that person may need—pain relief, escape from trauma, easing the sickness of withdrawal, or simply to just get high. Some who use opioids will develop addiction, which can make it difficult for a person to stop using drugs due to chemical changes in the brain even though they may recognize that continued drug use is harmful to them. I discuss the science of addiction.

Chapter 7: Treatment and Recovery

There are many paths to recovery. What treatment works for one person may not work for another. I discuss the choices facing someone who seeks to stop using drugs, beginning with the process of detoxification and continuing to treatment options from the gold standard of medication-assisted treatment with drugs like buprenorphine and methadone to abstinence preached by 12-step programs.

Chapter 8: Harm Reduction: Keeping People Alive

Driven by the mantra to "meet people where they are," harm reduction aims to reduce the negative consequences associated with drug use. I discuss harm reduction programs like syringe exchange, community naloxone, and overdose prevention centers, where people can use drugs under the watchful eyes of health care providers who can treat them if they overdose, provide aid for wounds, and guide them toward treatment if they desire it and other needed social services.

Chapter 9: The Harms of Stigma

The stigma of being an "addict" implies that person is to blame for their actions. Stigma causes people to hide their addiction, preventing them from seeking help. I discuss the dangers of stigma in its many forms, including language, and how we can avoid it.

Chapter 10: Ending the War on People/Hope for the Future
After 50 years of the War on Drugs, drugs are not only more dangerous than they have ever been, but they are also cheaper and more readily available. I discuss targeted law enforcement, decriminalization, legalization, and government regulation of a safe supply, as well as programs to address contributing causes of the epidemic, such as homelessness and lack of available mental health treatment.

PART THREE: ACTION

Key Points: 10 Lessons from This Book
This section shares the top take-home messages from this book.

Action Plan: A Seven-Point Agenda to Address the Crisis
Here I share six actions society can take to change the trajectory of the epidemic.

Glossary
The glossary features short explanations of terms and topics.

PART ONE

How to Recognize and Treat Overdose

CHAPTER 1

Overdose

Who Is at Risk

Today anyone who uses illicit opioids or pills not directly prescribed to them by a doctor is at risk for overdosing. This includes both experienced users and those using for the first time. Our current street drug supply is toxic, poison. No one who uses these drugs is safe.

I am the emergency medical services (EMS) representative on Connecticut's Overdose Fatality Review Panel. We meet regularly to review selected cases of people who have died of overdose. We receive a file on each person. The file describes who they were. We learn about their background, including their age, gender, race, family, education, and work history, as well as their medical and mental health history, including their experiences with substance use. The report specifies the circumstances and details of their death, including the autopsy and toxicology findings (fentanyl is almost always present). There are interviews with family members or friends, an assessment of their economic stability, descriptions

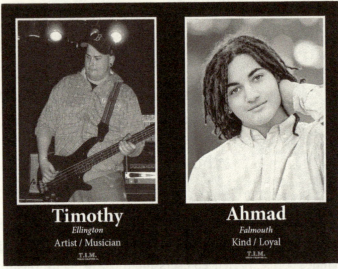
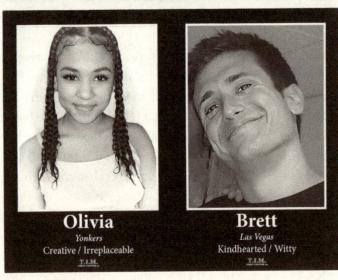

Today I Matter poster project honoring lost family and demonstrating they were much more than their drug problem

of their stressors, and an assessment of how well they were integrated into their community at the time of their death.

The cases, covered in these spare two- or three-page briefs, are soul crushing. We hear of the decedents' triumphs, struggles, and tragedies and their families' love for them. The cases show us the people they were, not society's stereotyped view of them. We see their missteps and stumbles and often the plain bad luck that jolted their paths—physical or mental abuse, the car accident or injury, the first opioid prescription, the death of a loved one, the mental health crisis, the failed rehab, unemployment, the divorce, the jail time, the homelessness. Reading the cases and already knowing their terrible end, you want to shout, "Stop that train! Please, please, someone help them!" It is like watching a high-speed car accident and not being able to do anything in the moment. You want to turn back time to take the steps needed to alter their fate.

As we discuss each brief, we look for missed opportunities. Was a mental health problem diagnosed too late? Should a health care provider have tapered the patient's opioid prescription instead of just cutting them off? Was the person who used ever offered methadone or buprenorphine, medications that have been proven to save lives by treating withdrawal symptoms and reducing opioid cravings? When they were kicked out of their sober house for using drugs, could somebody have offered them a bridge to a treatment program instead of throwing them out onto the street? Could housing assistance have helped them transition from their period of living in a tent in the woods? What happened that time they left the emergency department without being seen? Did the staff say something to them that caused them to walk out? Was naloxone in their parents' home the night they died? When I review the cases, I ask myself: Why did they start using drugs in the first place? Why did they continue to use? What could have been done to help them along the way? And why on this fatal occasion did they overdose and die?

It is a rare case that doesn't display multiple prominent risk factors. To get a grip on this epidemic, we must recognize what those risk factors are and their implications for drug use, drug use disorder, overdose, and overdose death. It is important to understand these factors and be vigilant in recognizing them in others, including our families and friends, and in ourselves. According to a recent study in the *American Journal of Public Health*, 42.4 percent of Americans know someone who died of a drug overdose, and one out of eight have had their lives disrupted by an overdose death. This crisis is not in a foreign land; it is in our towns and cities, in our neighborhoods and on our streets, and, for many, in our own homes.

OPIOID USE AND ADDICTION RISK FACTORS

An Opioid Prescription

The availability of opioids through a prescription increases the risk of drug use and, for some, subsequent addiction (opioid use disorder). For people who were first exposed to opioids through prescriptions, evidence shows that the risk of addiction elevates as soon as five days after beginning the prescription. In 2012 there were 81.3 opioid prescriptions for every 100 people in the country. Eleven states had more opioid prescriptions than people, led by Alabama with 143.8 prescriptions per 100 people. Fortunately, that has changed. By 2020, the number of prescriptions per 100 people in the United States was down to 43.2. Also, in many states, like Connecticut, prescribers are now limited to giving patients only a seven-day supply of opioid drugs for their initial prescription, unless they meet other requirements. The limit in Connecticut for minors is five days. Many doctors write prescriptions for even fewer days. This strategy appears to be working, as the rate of overdose death in young people is decreasing, suggesting fewer new people are becoming addicted through this gateway.

Other Access to Opioids

If friends, family members, or coworkers are using drugs and the drugs are readily available, the danger of misuse and addiction will rise. Some people's descents into drug use and addiction start not with their own prescription but with taking a pill from a friend, offered at a party or on the job to help with nagging pain. People using opioids prescribed to them should keep them safe from others and dispose of any leftover pills once they have stopped taking them. The increasing prevalence of counterfeit (fake) pills is another reason not to take pills from others. The offered Percocet could contain a lethal dose of fentanyl rather than the reliable dose of the advertised product you would expect from a pharmaceutical pill.

History of Substance Use

Those who have used other substances, such as marijuana or cocaine, may be less reluctant to try opioids than someone who has never used substances. There is much debate about whether marijuana is a gateway drug. For the most part, I don't believe it is. I smoked marijuana in my college years in the late 1970s, but I would have run if anyone had offered me heroin, which I associated with dirty needles, ugly tattoos, and death in a dark alley. What is not debatable is that people with experience misusing prescription opioid drugs such as oxycontin are at a higher risk of transitioning to heroin or fentanyl, which are similar chemical substances but cheaper, stronger, and more readily available on the black market than legitimate prescription pills. As mentioned earlier and as I will detail later, many of the pills sold today on the black market that look just like brand name pills are fake containing an unknown amount of fentanyl rather than the prescription drug they purport to be.

Age at First Use

The earlier someone begins using substances, the more likely they are to develop substance use problems. Because young people's brains are malleable and not fully formed, they are more easily rewired by opioids' effects on the brain's reward pathways. Research published in *Pediatrics* in November 2015 found that when prescribed an opioid before their senior year in high school, people with no drug use history and who strongly disapproved of others smoking marijuana had a 33 percent greater risk of engaging in harmful opioid use later in life than those who had no opioid prescription.

Adverse Childhood Experiences

People with adverse childhood experiences (ACEs) are at higher risk of later substance use and addiction. These experiences include physical, emotional, or sexual abuse as well as physical or emotional neglect. They also include growing up in a dysfunctional household, which is defined as living with someone with mental illness, having a relative in jail, having a mother who is treated violently, the presence of substance use in the home, or a history of divorce. These risk factors are combined to create an "ACE score." The higher the ACE score, the higher the risk of drug misuse. One study found that for each point in the ACE score, a person's chance of early illicit drug use increased twofold to fourfold.

Mental Health

There is a known link between substance use and mental health. According to the Centers for Disease Control and

Prevention's (CDC's) State Unintentional Drug Overdose Reporting System (SUDORS), an estimated 25.4 percent of people who die of overdose have an underlying mental health concern. For many with undiagnosed mental health issues, drugs help treat underlying issues such as depression, anxiety, and post-traumatic stress disorder (PTSD), and this can encourage their continued use despite the dangers.

Personality

People with impulsivity or thrill-seeking traits are at increased risk to use drugs. Their lack of hesitation may propel them into making choices they might not have made upon due consideration.

Genetics

A 2023 National Institutes of Health study confirmed what researchers have long surmised: that certain inheritable genes are commonly linked with both substance use and mental health issues. Some of the genes involve the brain's dopamine or reward system, which can be hijacked by drug use, as I will explain in the chapter on addiction. Having any of these genes does not guarantee that someone will develop addiction or substance use disorder, but combined with environmental influences, they can make substance use disorder more likely in one person than in another subject to the same influences. For one person a night of drinking alcohol and snorting a line of cocaine can lead to nothing more than a bad hangover, but for another, it can start them on an unanticipated road to addiction and eventual death from drug use.

Gender

Males are at higher risk of substance use disorder than females because they are more likely to use opioids than women. In 2021, 70 percent of those who died of overdose in the country were male. In Connecticut, 72 percent of EMS-reported overdoses in 2022 were male. These numbers have remained remarkably consistent over the years. Once a person begins using, there are no gender differences in who will develop addiction.

Age

The age group hit hardest by overdose deaths is those 35–44 years, followed by 45–54 and then 25–34. That said, overdose deaths, particularly in the age of fentanyl, include infants and senior citizens. According to the Connecticut Office of the Child Advocate, since 2020, there have been 11 fentanyl-caused deaths among infants and toddlers in the state, with many more resuscitated with naloxone. These deaths are attributed to the young children accidentally getting into poorly secured drug caches or poorly sanitized surfaces where drugs may have been used or packaged. Among the elderly, overdose deaths quadrupled between 2002 and 2021, reflecting the general rise in overdose deaths. In 2021, overdose rates in those 65 and over increased 28 percent, the largest percentage increase among age groups. As the baby boomer generation is now attaining retirement age, those who experimented with drugs when young may be less averse than the previous generation (the Silent Generation) to using drugs. Older people may also be less able to sustain the superpowered opioids like fentanyl.

Occupation

Those engaged in industries such as construction, extraction (mining, oil, and gas extraction), and food preparation have higher proportional rates for fatal overdose than other occupations. This could be due to availability of drugs in these professions, higher risk of injury from physical labor, and lack of sick leave necessitating a person perform that labor despite injury in order to get paid. When I ask my patients how they got started using opioids, it is not uncommon for someone to say they got hurt on a construction site and a coworker gave them pills to help with their pain so they could keep working.

OVERDOSE AND DEATH RISKS

Polydrug Use

Using more than one drug at the same time—known as *polydrug use*—can also increase the risk of overdose. Combine an opioid, which is a sedative, with other sedatives like benzodiazepines or alcohol, and there is increased risk for unconsciousness and depressed or absent breathing. Using opioids with stimulants like cocaine or methamphetamine can also exacerbate risk. Stimulants can cause vasoconstriction, a narrowing of the body's blood vessels, and an accelerated heart rate, requiring the body to use more oxygen; the opioids, however, are simultaneously depressing the body's ability to obtain oxygen, leading to decreased oxygen intake and death. Many users frequently use both opioids and stimulants to find the proper equilibrium between being too up or too down. In 2021, 32.3 percent of all fatal overdoses contained both fentanyl and a stimulant, although it is not clear the role each drug played in any individual death as opposed to merely being present in the user's system. Opioids are more likely to kill by overdose in the moment by stopping a person's breathing, while stimulants may kill over the longer term with the damage they wreak on the body, particularly by overstressing the cardiovascular system.

Injecting Opioids

Injecting directly into the bloodstream provides the quickest and most powerful delivery of opioids compared with other routes of exposure (snorting, smoking, ingesting, etc.). The bioavailability—the amount of drug that reaches the brain—is highest with intravenous delivery. The stereotype of the drug user dying with the needle still in their arm is based in fact. The drug can hit the brain while the user is still slowly pushing the syringe plunger forward, causing them to lose consciousness before even finishing their shot. People who inject often start taking opioid pills orally and then progress to crushing the pills and snorting the powder for a stronger effect, and finally to injecting. In addition to the risk of sudden death, injection also poses the risk of transmission of diseases such as AIDS and hepatitis C when needles are shared.

Abstinence

Years ago, I thought many of my resuscitated overdose patients were lying when they said things to me like: "I don't use drugs anymore." "I just slipped up." "I haven't used in months." "I just got out of rehab." "This is the first time in two years I have used." When I started reading about drug use, I began to understand the truth behind many of their statements. Only a small amount of opioid may be needed to get a novice or opioid-naive person high. That same person, should they continue to use, will soon need greater amounts of the drug to achieve the same high. People who use opioids regularly develop tolerance to the opioid, sometimes in a matter of days. When tolerance develops, a higher dose is needed to achieve the same effects. The body has adjusted to the opioid. This cycle of needing more and more opioids to achieve the same effect continues. When someone stops using opioids, their tolerance drops. If a person who is used to doing three bags of heroin at a time uses three bags when they return to using opioids after an extended absence, they will likely overdose as their body is no longer tolerant to such a high dose. A dose of two milligrams of fentanyl may be lethal to one person, whereas another with greater tolerance might require ten milligrams to achieve a fatal dose. Those with lowered tolerance include patients recently discharged from treatment, those recently released from incarceration, and those who have undergone a self-imposed period of abstinence. Many prisons and drug treatment facilities now routinely give people naloxone, the opioid antidote, on their discharge. Unfortunately, these same three groups of recent users are likely to hide their drug use from others and will often use alone with no one to monitor them for overdose.

Prior Nonfatal Overdose

Not everyone who overdoses is going to overdose again. Nearly all opioid overdoses are unintentional. A study in Massachusetts, however, showed that 10 percent of people who received naloxone from EMS for an overdose were dead within a year. Overdosing is unpleasant, and so is resuscitation with naloxone, but if people use illicit street drugs, the risk of overdose and death will be there.

Using Alone

The number one risk factor for dying of a fatal overdose is using opioids alone. Ninety-one percent of all fatal opioid overdoses in 2021 were unwitnessed. As a paramedic I am often dispatched on "welfare checks" for people who have not been seen for some time or whose neighbor has complained of a smell coming from an apartment. The supervisor lets us in. We find the patient dead on the floor or slumped across a couch or bed. It is not uncommon to find an unopened box of naloxone on scene along with discharge papers from a treatment facility or prison release. Naloxone won't work if there is no one to administer it.

One Use Can Kill

A person doesn't have to be addicted to opioids to accidentally overdose on them. While people addicted to opioids are at a higher risk for overdose because they use more often than people who are not addicted, no one is safe. The unpredictable ingredients and strength of current street drugs pose great danger. One illicit pill or bag of powder—ingested, snorted, smoked, or injected—can kill.

Opportunity for Intervention

According to the CDC, in 2021, 65 percent of people who died of fatal overdose had a potential opportunity for intervention before their deaths, including interaction with mental health or substance use treatment, recent release from prison, or someone in the area who could have delivered naloxone had they known the person was overdosing in a nearby room or another accessible space. **Know the aforementioned risk factors, and be on guard.**

Bread

There are three loaves of bread sticking out of a paper bag in the passenger seat of the car. I recognize them from the bakery on Park Street where people pick up fresh, long loaves of the crusty pan de agua (water bread) hot out of the ovens beginning when the shop opens at six. It is now eleven on this brisk November day, and the bread, like the young man who bought them, is cold. We pull the man out of the parked car, lay him down on the pavement in the apartment building's isolated rear lot, and begin CPR. Now a woman screams when she recognizes the man. Children run out the back door of the building. The older onlookers try to shield the children's view. We work to resuscitate him for thirty minutes and then five more on the short trip to the hospital, but the straight line on the monitor never changes.

CHAPTER 2

How to Recognize Overdose

Every citizen should learn to quickly recognize an opioid overdose and take the necessary steps to reverse the overdose and save the life of a loved one or a stranger.

WHAT TO LOOK FOR

Unconsciousness, slow or absent breathing, and pinpoint pupils are the hallmarks of an opioid overdose.

HOW OPIOIDS WORK

Opioids act on our central nervous system. Opioids include common prescription pills such as oxycodone and Percocet as well as the illicit drugs heroin and fentanyl. At normal doses, opioids produce pleasure and pain relief. At higher doses, opioids depress consciousness and reduce respirations.

Opioids kill by stopping a person from breathing enough to sustain life and producing cardiac arrest. When we breathe, the incoming oxygen is absorbed into tiny air sacs in our lungs called alveoli. There the oxygen is absorbed into

HOW TO RECOGNIZE OVERDOSE

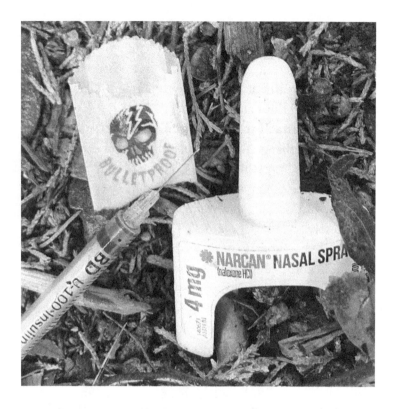

our bloodstream, where it is carried to the heart and then pumped (via arteries) throughout our body to our organs and brain, nourishing our cells. The waste products of the exchange—carbon dioxide—are returned by the veins to our lungs. Back in the alveoli, the carbon dioxide is expelled when we breathe out. If we get too much carbon dioxide in our blood, our body increases its respiratory rate to expel the gas. Our body is programmed to help us maintain the proper equilibrium. Oxygen in. Carbon dioxide out. Without thinking about it, we breathe at a natural rhythm, rate, and depth. Opioids can affect this balance.

Opioids attach to the receptors in our brain, which control breathing. As the receptors become overloaded with opioids, breathing slows. Normally, as the carbon dioxide in the blood starts to rise, the body is triggered to breathe, but opioids can hinder this response or block it completely.

People become cyanotic as the oxygen in their bloodstream becomes depleted. Cyanosis, a blue or purplish discoloration of the skin, is seen first in the fingers and near the lips. As oxygen decreases, carbon dioxide rises to dangerous levels. While many people may lose consciousness and have slowed breathing, if they receive enough oxygen to maintain organ function, they can survive until the opioid wears off.

When breathing slows to a critical level or stops in an opioid overdose, a person becomes hypoxic. Hypoxia means lack of oxygen. The heart will continue to pump blood to the brain, but with each beat, the amount of oxygen in the circulating blood becomes even further depleted, and each beat itself becomes less powerful until the hypoxic heart, now starved of oxygen, stops altogether.

SIGNS OF OPIOID USE

Pinpoint Pupils

One of the telltale signs of opioid use is constricted or pinpoint pupils, also known as *miosis*. The pupil is the dot in the center of your eye. Opioids act on the eyes' pupillary response. While there are many factors that affect pupillary response, if a person with a history of opioid use has pinpoint pupils, they are likely under the influence of opioids. Most other drugs and alcohol dilate or enlarge pupils. Pinpoint pupils alone is only a sign of possible opioid use, not overdose. An overdose begins when the drug exceeds its intended effects and impairs consciousness and breathing.

Stupor

Opioids produce euphoria, intense feelings of happiness and well-being. They can also produce stupor, a deep lethargy and near unconsciousness that requires stimulation to be aroused from. It is not uncommon to find people on opioids to be "on the nod." They are breathing and may be standing or sitting with their heads slumped forward as if they have nodded off to sleep. For some, this depressed consciousness state is not an overdose but often the intended outcome, the feeling the user sought when taking the drug. People on the nod are still breathing adequately and often can be roused with a simple shake.

SIGNS OF OPIOID OVERDOSE

Unconsciousness

Depressed consciousness, which can precede or accompany decreased breathing, may lead to unconsciousness. One of the dangers of unconsciousness is that a person may accidentally block their airway with their tongue or bend their neck so much that it prevents them from taking in air. Snoring may be heard from an overdosed patient whose tongue partially blocks their airway. Sometimes people in the nodding position fall forward into a praying or frog-like position, burying their heads in a couch, a bed, or another object or bending their neck until they accidentally suffocate, too unresponsive to recognize their body's need to breathe. Opioids can also depress the gag reflex, making it hard for a person who is still breathing to protect their lungs from secretions and vomit, which can cause them to choke to death. Others who don't choke may develop aspiration pneumonia if these secretions get into their lungs, damaging the alveoli, introducing bacteria into the lungs, and decreasing the available surface for gas exchange.

Decreased Respirations/Cyanosis/Apnea

When opioids cause respirations (breathing) to become inadequate, cyanosis develops. A bluish tint to the skin is soon visible. Overdose can present as gurgling, snoring, or irregular, shallow, or eventually absent breathing, called *apnea*. We normally breathe between 12 and 20 times a minute. If someone is breathing only 2 to 4 times a minute, and their breathing is labored or gasping, we call this *agonal breathing*. It can also be called a death rattle. Witnesses often recall having heard the victim snoring or making loud rattling noises, and only after the victim was found dead did the witness realize they had been overdosing at the time. Once a person has stopped breathing, death will follow unless respirations can be restored within minutes. Sometimes in an overdose, a person's airway can become occluded (blocked off) by the glottis, a piece of tissue that guards the trachea, our airway, to prevent food from entering the lungs when we swallow. An occluded glottis causes pressure to build up in the chest. The pressure can damage the alveoli, creating a pink frothy liquid known as *pulmonary edema*. A pink foam cone on the mouth and nose is not uncommon in patients who are found dead of opioid overdose.

Seizure

Overdoses of the synthetic opioid fentanyl can sometimes make it appear that the person is having a seizure, with the fentanyl causing the person's muscles to become rigid as muscles do in the tonic phase of a seizure. This can prevent the chest from expanding and lead to suffocation. Naloxone will immediately stop the rigidity. It is believed this fentanyl-caused rigidity may also be the reason a patient's glottis closes, leading to near-immediate respiratory arrest.

Opioid Packaging and Paraphernalia

External clues that can indicate an unconscious person has suffered an opioid overdose include the presence of syringes or paraphernalia, such as small plastic bags, drug packaging, a bottle cap, or a cooker in the room. Needle marks and scabbing may be present on their arms, including the crook of the elbow or the hands and forearms, where their veins are close to the skin. Not everyone who overdoses on opioids, however, injects their opioids. Many overdoses are caused by inhalation, ingestion, or smoking, which offer different clues. For those who smoke opioids, aluminum foil with black residue can indicate recent drug use. Straws or rolled-up bills may indicate the person snorted the drugs, especially if powder is visible nearby. Still, signs of drug use may not be near the overdosed patient. Most users, particularly if they live with non-users, go to great lengths to hide their use, so absence of paraphernalia does not mean absence of use.

EFFECTS OF ROUTES OF ADMINISTRATION ON OVERDOSE

Opioids can be consumed in several ways—taken orally as a pill, snorted as a powder, smoked by heating on aluminum foil and inhaling the vapors, absorbed transdermally (through the skin) by specially designed patches, or injected into a muscle or vein. They can also be inserted into the rectum in an act known as "boofing."

Potency

Injection into a vein provides the most rapid onset, while swallowing a pill provides a much slower onset as the drug must be digested and then slowly make its way into the circulation, which carries the opioid up to the brain. The bioavailability of the drug—the amount that gets metabolized, or its useful strength—is 100 percent when used intravenously. The bioavailability of a drug is much lower when taken orally. Oxycodone, for instance, has a bioavailability of only 60 percent when taken orally, while morphine has a bioavailability of only 33 percent when taken orally. Oxycodone's bioavailability increases to 77 percent when snorted. That is why people transition from swallowing pills to crushing and snorting them to injecting them—so they can achieve greater potency or effect.

Time of Onset

Those who use intravenously can sometimes stop breathing before they have even finished injecting their full dose if they get an unexpectedly strong product. Snorting and smoking have a slightly longer onset. Ingesting a pill will result in a much longer onset, and transdermal patches may take up to 24 hours to work. People who have used too strong of a dose may remain alert if someone stimulates them with some kind of external stimulation, but when they sit or are left alone, their breathing may slow and then stop.

HOW TO RESPOND TO AN OVERDOSE

When you suspect an unconscious person is suffering from an opioid overdose, the first thing to do is try to stimulate them. Often, stimulation alone will restore breathing and consciousness. Shake the person's shoulder while calling their name. If that does not immediately work, rub your knuckles hard against their sternum (breastbone). This is painful but can elicit a response. While stimulation alone can restore adequate breathing and consciousness, people may continue to drift off and should still be monitored and stimulated as necessary if their breathing again slows. If you can lay the person on their side, do so. Whether they are on the ground or sitting up, make certain their head is tilted back so they are not blocking their airway.

To determine if a person is breathing, look for chest rise or check to see if any air is coming out of the person's nose or mouth. If you are uncertain if they are breathing, you must check for a pulse. A pulse indicates whether the heart is beating well enough to provide or perfuse the body with oxygen. When the heart beats, it generates a flow of blood through the arteries to the cells and can be felt on the wrist, upper arm, groin, and neck. The neck is the most accessible place to feel the pulse, and you can usually feel it even if the person's blood pressure is too low to palpate at the other locations. Place your fingers against the side of the person's neck. Do not press on the trachea or front of the neck; go at least an inch to the side. Try it now on yourself or a friend. Feel it? In some people, the pulse in the neck at the carotid artery is so prevalent you can even see it throbbing. In others, particularly people with short, fat necks, it is harder to feel. It is okay if you can't find it on everyone. I have been a paramedic for thirty years, and there are still some people whose carotid pulses I cannot feel even when they are talking to me.

If a person is not breathing and you can't feel a pulse, you should start CPR, which I will explain in the next chapter.

If a person has a pulse and is breathing adequately but is not responsive, roll them onto their side to prevent them from choking if they vomit.

If a person has a pulse but is breathing inadequately despite stimulation, this person should receive naloxone, which I will also describe in the next chapter.

In any case, call 911 as soon as possible.

Wrestler

"I can't wake him up!" the mother says as we come into the bedroom. Her voice and hands are shaking. "He was fine when I went out for groceries. Now he won't respond." She is crying. "Honey! Honey!" she says.

Her son lies limply back on his bed, breathing only about four times a minute. He is wearing a New York Knicks jersey and has a few days' growth of beard. There is a long scar on his shoulder. He looks to be about 20 years old. "What drugs does he use?" I ask as I check his pupils. They are pinpoint. "Pills? Heroin?"

"No," she says. "He doesn't use drugs. He just came home yesterday from college for the holiday. He doesn't even drink anymore."

My partner hands me the bag-valve-mask. I place the mask over the young man's mouth, tilt his head back, and squeeze the bag, sending oxygen into his lungs. When he does not respond after a few breaths, I have my partner breathe for him while I put an IV in his arm. Our monitor shows his oxygen saturation is low and his carbon dioxide is dangerously high. I take the naloxone out of my med kit, draw up a small amount in a syringe, and slowly push it through the IV. In a matter of moments, the boy's respirations pick up, and his carbon dioxide drops as his oxygen rises. We no longer have to breathe for him. Two minutes later his eyes open, and he looks about with a start. "It's okay," I say. "Rest, you overdosed. We had to give you naloxone. You're not in trouble."

He swears and lays his head back down. "I just used half a bag," he says. "I can't believe this."

"Rest," I say. "It's okay."

He tells me the story. He had just broken up with his girlfriend, and when he met the guy who used to sell him drugs before he went to rehab after his junior year, he let his guard down.

While my partner helps him find his shoes, I go into the hallway, where his mom is still with the police officer. "He's fine," I say. "He's alert and breathing. We had to give him some naloxone."

"He overdosed?" she says. "That can't be!"

"His pupils were pinpoint. He wasn't breathing well. We gave him a little naloxone and he came around. He's talking to us now. You should have naloxone in your house. Do you know where to get it?"

"But he doesn't use anymore. He went to rehab. He's been clean for almost two years. I was just talking to him. He's been doing great."

She is not the first mother who has been shocked to find her child has overdosed. I explain to her that she should not be upset with her son. Two years of not using is something to be proud of. Relapse is not unexpected. If he made it two years, he can do it again, and maybe even longer, but she needs to have naloxone in the house just in case. I tell her how to recognize an overdose and where to get naloxone and how to use it. Then I take her in to see her son. She sits beside him on the bed and hugs him.

"I'm sorry, Mom," he says.

"It's okay," she says, tearfully. "I'm not mad at you. You've been through a lot. You mean everything to me."

On the wall there is a picture of him in a wrestling singlet and a medal around his neck. His parents are standing proudly on either side of him.

CHAPTER 3

Naloxone

Naloxone, an opioid antagonist, reverses the effects of opioids on the respiratory system. Because naloxone has a stronger affinity for the brain's breathing receptors (the mu receptors) than opioids do, it knocks opioids off the receptors and enables a person to resume breathing. It does not have to knock all the opioids off to work, however. It is estimated that knocking even 50 percent of the opioids off the receptors is sufficient for a person to breathe sustainably. As long as a person's heart has not stopped, naloxone will usually reverse an opioid overdose if given in time. Naloxone does not work on nonopioid drugs, such as benzodiazepines, cocaine, methamphetamines, or alcohol, but since these drugs are often used in combination with opioids, the naloxone will reverse the opioid contribution to the overdose—the slowing or cessation of breathing, the symptom most likely to cause death.

WHO CARRIES NALOXONE?

Naloxone is now available to the public without a prescription. Years ago, only paramedics, the highest level of

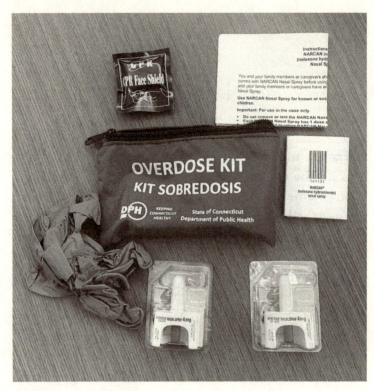

Contents of naloxone overdose kit

emergency medical technician (EMT), were able to administer naloxone outside the hospital. Today, naloxone is carried by most first responders, including police, firefighters, and basic-level EMTs, as well as members of the public. In Connecticut in 2023, in 21 percent of all overdoses where 911 was called, naloxone was first given by a public person before first responders arrived. In 58 percent of overdoses, naloxone was administered by the public or first responders such as police and firefighters before the EMS ambulance arrived. This does not include the unknown number of overdoses where people successfully administered naloxone to overdose victims and 911 was not called.

HOW IS NALOXONE GIVEN?

Naloxone can be given in three forms: intranasally (IN) by nasal spray, intramuscularly (IM) by injection with a needle through the skin and into the muscle, or intravenously (IV) through a needle/catheter into a blood vein. Naloxone works fastest when given intravenously, but this requires a medical professional to first establish IV access.

Intranasal Spray

Intranasal spray is the most common form of naloxone available to the public and the easiest to use, but it is the slowest to take effect. Its brand names include Narcan and Kloxxado, which accounted for 96 percent of all prescription naloxone products sold in 2021. They are FDA approved and specifically formulated for intranasal administration. Intranasal naloxone comes in a blister pack. The Narcan device contains 4 mg of naloxone in just 0.1 cc of fluid and has the same bioavailability as 2 mg injected into the muscle. The device is intuitive and quite simple to use. If you have ever self-administered a nasal spray to relieve decongestion, you can administer naloxone spray. A research study found that 90 percent of untrained users were able to administer intranasal naloxone successfully.

To administer naloxone, tear the device out of the blister pack. Tilt the person's head back. Hold your thumb on the bottom of the device plunger, and insert the nozzle into the nose (either nostril). Press the plunger with your thumb. That's it. A small note of caution: Be careful not to press the plunger until the device is in the nose to prevent accidental discharge. Each device holds only one spray.

The package instructions call for naloxone to be redosed every two to three minutes until the patient responds. For many laypeople, "patient responds" means the patient wakes up, but to professional rescuers, "responding" means the patient is able to breathe again on their own. Consciousness usually follows restored breathing, often several minutes later. Stimulation will help the person regain both breathing and consciousness sooner.

If you do have to administer a second dose, use the second nostril. For those inexperienced in witnessing opioid overdose, it may be difficult to judge time. Ten seconds can seem like a minute, one minute like five. It is understandable that someone might give the second dose before two or three minutes have elapsed, particularly if the person is blue. Professional rescuers have the ability to breathe for unresponsive patients with a bag-valve-mask device. The person is getting oxygen so the situation is now less critical. It is just a matter of waiting the necessary minutes for the naloxone to kick in so the person can begin breathing on their own. Bystanders rarely provide the less effective mouth-to-mouth or a face-shield-to-mouth breathing, particularly if the overdosed person is a stranger. The situation is more dire for them as the patient is likely still not getting the full oxygen they need. I have been on many scenes where bystanders have quickly emptied all the naloxone they have into a patient in hopes that it will restore them to breathing sooner.

Until the overdose victim is conscious, be certain to place the person on their side in what is known as the recovery position. This will help protect the person from choking if they vomit. **Patients who are dependent on opioids may vomit as the naloxone wipes the opioids out of their system.** A person dependent on opioids needs to maintain a certain level of opioid in their system to avoid getting sick. Naloxone can put them into precipitated withdrawal, causing nausea, vomiting, sweating, and body aches, among other unpleasant symptoms. While giving too many doses of naloxone may worsen withdrawal symptoms, these symptoms are less severe than a person not breathing.

Kloxxado contains 8 mg of naloxone in comparison to Narcan's 4 mg. Many argue that that is too much and will more easily lead to severe withdrawal in patients addicted to opioids. A recent study found this to be the case. There was no difference in survival benefit between the 4 mg and 8 mg devices, and the 8 mg device produced more withdrawal symptoms. Still, if an 8 mg device is all you have, go ahead and use it. A vomiting patient is better than one not breathing. Another drug on the market that has just been approved is nalmefene, sold as Opvee, which is similar to naloxone but lasts much longer. There is debate about the need for such a drug and the fear that it will also increase withdrawal symptoms. Pharmaceutical companies argue that these more powerful opioid antidotes are needed to contend with the stronger fentanyl, but this has not been proven and remains a pharmaceutical talking point. In Connecticut, nalmefene is not approved for use by emergency responders. The FDA has also approved a 3 mg nasal naloxone called RiVive, which is manufactured by a nonprofit. This is acceptable for use by EMS and is less expensive than the other brands.

The atomizer, a second type of intranasal spray device that is not FDA approved but is still commonly used, is more complicated to administer. The atomizer was the first intranasal device we used in EMS before the single-unit devices were available, and it is still preferred by many in EMS due to its ability to be titrated—that is, to administer the smallest required dosage initially and increase it as needed rather than having to give the full dose in one spray. This type of intranasal spray involves screwing a prefilled vial of naloxone into a tube and then attaching a cone-shaped atomizer to the end of the tube. The vial contains 2 mg of naloxone in 2 cc of fluid (as compared with Narcan's 4 mg in 0.1 cc). Its bioavailability is the equivalent of 0.4 mg injected into the muscle, and it is less concentrated than the naloxone in the single dose nasal sprays. **To administer it, insert the atomizer into one nostril, push the vial to the halfway point, and then switch nostrils and push the remaining amount from the vial (1 cc).** The naloxone will not work unless the atomizer is attached. You must also push briskly or the fluid will not turn into a spray of the tiny particles necessary to pass through the brain's blood barrier and displace the opioids from the brain's receptors. It is not unusual to see some of the naloxone draining back out of the nose. While containing far more fluid, this device contains far fewer active ingredients than the nasal spray. Nevertheless, it has proven effective and is also less likely to induce withdrawal. The downsides are that it may take longer to work, and it is not as intuitive as the Narcan device. Research studies have also shown it is difficult for untrained users to successfully deliver naloxone through this method. If you obtain this type of naloxone, familiarize yourself with it beforehand. Watch a video from the manufacturers or on YouTube, or take the device out and study it.

Intramuscular Naloxone

There are two main types of intramuscular injection—an auto-injector and a syringe and vial.

The first auto-injector, Evzio, was so expensive (over a thousand dollars per dose) that it has been discontinued. It was modeled after Epipens, which are used for anaphylactic reactions. An auto-injector involves removing the device from its case, pulling off a safety guard, placing the auto-injector against a patient's outer thigh (the upper part of the leg), and pressing firmly for several seconds while holding in place. You can go through the clothes if you have to. The Evzio contained 2 mg of naloxone. A new auto-injector on the market called Zimhi has 5 mg. As with Kloxxado, many feel that this is an excessive dose at more than two and a half times the most powerful dose a paramedic would deliver intramuscularly. **To administer, twist off the needle cap. Press the needle into the outer thigh. Push the plunger until it clicks, and hold it in for at least two seconds before removing it from the leg.** Again, it is a good idea with any naloxone device to review a video tutorial.

The syringe and vial method is the least expensive and is often preferred by people who use drugs (particularly IV drug users who are comfortable with needles). Intramuscular naloxone works quicker than intranasal and has the fewest side effects due to its lower dose of 0.4 mg. It is the first-line medicine (after oxygen) used in New York City's safe injection sites. The medicine comes in a small vial (0.4 mg of naloxone in 1 cc of fluid). **To administer, pop the top off the vial. Insert the syringe through the vial's rubber top, turn the vial upside down, and pull back on the plunger until the vial is empty. Insert the syringe needle into a large muscle, either in the thigh (preferred due to the presence of more blood vessels to carry the drug to the heart) or the upper arm. Push the plunger forward until it stops, and then remove the syringe.**

After giving any type of naloxone, always stay with the person until first responders arrive.

ADMINISTER NALOXONE OR CALL 911 FIRST?

If you are alone with the overdose victim and have naloxone, administer it, and then call 911. Get professional rescuers on the way. If someone is with you, have them call 911 while you administer the naloxone. There is some controversy as to the proper order of calling 911 versus giving naloxone first. My advice is to use common sense if you are alone. If the naloxone is in your hand, administer it, and then call 911. If you have to search all over the house for the naloxone, call 911 first and then find and administer the naloxone.

TREATMENT FOR PEOPLE WHO ARE NOT BREATHING OR MAY NOT HAVE A PULSE

Determining whether an overdose victim is breathing is much easier than finding a pulse. If their chest isn't moving and no air is coming out of their nose or mouth after waiting approximately 15–30 seconds, feel their neck for a pulse. If the person has a pulse and is not breathing, start rescue breathing if you are comfortable with it. If the person is breathing, there is no need to check for a pulse. In order to breathe, a person's heart must be beating.

Rescue breathing involves putting the person on their back and tilting their head backward to open their airway. If you have a plastic breath barrier or mask, use it for your protection. Pinch their nose closed, and give one breath every five seconds. Watch the chest for rise, which indicates air is going into the lungs. If you cannot find a pulse and the person is still not breathing, assume they do not have a pulse and start CPR.

CPR (CARDIOPULMONARY RESUSCITATION)

In addition to carrying naloxone, you should learn cardiopulmonary resuscitation, or CPR. Classes are widely available both in person and online. You never know when CPR might come in handy. To perform it, put your hands over the center of the person's chest, with the heel of one hand against the chest bone (sternum) and the other hand on top of your first hand. Keeping your elbows straight, put your shoulders above your hands and begin compressing to a depth of two inches. After each push, allow the chest to recoil, and don't move your hands. Keep them on the chest. Compress at a rate of 120 times a minute. If you cannot remember that, press to the beat of the Bee Gees' "Stayin' Alive." If you do not want to pause to give rescue breaths, it is okay to continue to just give compressions. The up-and-down movement on the chest actually provides passive ventilation through the compression of the chest and lungs, allowing the unconscious person to take in some oxygen and expel carbon dioxide.

Most advanced medical professionals do not give naloxone to people who are in cardiac arrest. Naloxone will not restore breathing if the heart is stopped. But it is okay for laypeople to administer naloxone on the chance that the person still has a pulse, even if it is too hard to feel. Compressions are often the stimulation needed to rouse someone (not in cardiac arrest) from overdose. Provide chest compressions if you are not sure whether the person has a pulse.

RESPONSE TO NALOXONE

The instructions for naloxone call for it to be given every two to three minutes until the person is breathing on their own.

After you have given naloxone, continue to stimulate the person. This may speed up their visible response to the drug. In an emergency, it is sometimes difficult to judge time. It is important to remember that restoring adequate breathing is the goal, not consciousness, which usually follows minutes after adequate breathing has been restored. **If the person is breathing adequately and they are no longer cyanotic, even if they have not returned to full consciousness, no additional naloxone needs to be given.** These additional doses may put the patient, if they are dependent on opioids, into withdrawal.

PRECIPITATED WITHDRAWAL

If a person is dependent on opioids, naloxone may put the person into opioid withdrawal, characterized by symptoms such as sweating, nausea, rapid heart rate, vomiting, diarrhea, confusion, and agitation. This is why professional rescuers only give the smallest amount of naloxone necessary to restore breathing. (We are able to slowly titrate the naloxone to effect because we are able to breathe for the patient using bag-valve masks until the naloxone has had time to knock the opioid off the brain receptors.) Laypeople should not let the fear of putting a person into withdrawal cause them to withhold naloxone, however. **Withhold additional naloxone once the person has resumed effective breathing on their own.**

DRUGS RESISTANT TO NALOXONE

If the person is under the effects of another substance such as alcohol, a benzodiazepine, or an additive such as xylazine, they may not return to consciousness, but as long as they are breathing, the immediate catastrophe has been avoided. It is estimated that 80 percent of people who suffered synthetic opioid overdoses in 2016 were also using another drug or alcohol.

As previously mentioned, **naloxone only works on opioids.** It does not work on other categories of drugs or alcohol, but if an opioid is involved, that opioid is likely the chief cause of the depressed respirations, and naloxone will work to reverse that by knocking the opioid off the brain receptors that control breathing. The opioid, particularly if fentanyl is involved, is the drug most likely to cause death, and naloxone will prevent that death if given in time.

POST-RESUSCITATION

Reassure a person coming back to consciousness from an overdose. Speak quietly. Tell them they overdosed and that you gave them naloxone because their breathing was inadequate.

Do not be judgmental. They are likely to be confused from lack of oxygen. Help orient them by repeating what happened, telling them where they are, and reassuring them that they are with someone who cares about them. Do not be surprised if the person denies drug use. In Connecticut, 27 percent of patients resuscitated with naloxone denied use of any drugs at all on 911 calls, while 24 percent refused to say what drugs they had used. Denial may be a reflex to avoid getting in trouble or to defend from being judged negatively. Continue to be reassuring, and **stay with the person until professional help arrives**.

Naloxone Risks

You cannot overdose on naloxone. Naloxone does not get you high. Nor can you become addicted to it or develop a tolerance for it. If you overdose again, naloxone will be no less effective the second time. If the person is not on opioids, naloxone will not harm them. There is some speculation that in rare cases, naloxone can cause pulmonary edema—that is, fluid in the lungs—but others believe naloxone just uncovers pulmonary edema caused by damage to the alveoli due to a closed glottis during overdose. Bottom line: if you suspect an opioid overdose and that person has inadequate or absent breathing, do not hesitate to administer naloxone.

Things Not to Do

In EMS, we often encounter friends, families, and bystanders using unscientific home remedies to attempt to revive the overdosed person. Laying the person in a cold bath, dousing them with water, or putting ice in their pants are among the most common. While these actions may achieve some stimulation effect, if the person does not respond to initial stimulation, they are unlikely to respond to these measures, which have no effect on breathing mechanisms. Also, do not pour liquid into an unconscious person's mouth. Some incorrectly believe milk will counteract the overdose, but an unconscious person has no way to protect their airway. The liquid will choke them or permit the fluids to enter their lungs, damaging their alveoli and impairing their ability to exchange oxygen and carbon dioxide.

WHO SHOULD CARRY NALOXONE?

In 2018, US surgeon general Dr. Jerome Adams issued a rare advisory (the first in 13 years) urging Americans to carry naloxone. Adams, whose brother was serving a 10-year term for stealing $200 to support his addiction, stated, "Knowing how to use naloxone and keeping it within reach can save a life." He cited research showing that overdose deaths decrease in neighborhoods when community members are trained in the use of naloxone.

If anyone in your household is using opioids, either with a prescription or illicitly, or has a history of opioid use, you should have naloxone in your medicine cabinet. Eighty-seven percent of Connecticut's overdose deaths occur in a residence. You should also consider carrying naloxone with you when you travel, keeping it in a purse, a backpack, or the glove box of your car. If you encounter someone suffering an opioid overdose and use it to save their life, you will be glad you kept it handy, just as you would if a stranger carrying naloxone discovered someone you love overdosing in a public place and saved their life.

The broader the naloxone availability, the more lives will be saved.

WHERE CAN NALOXONE BE OBTAINED?

Intranasal naloxone is now available for over-the-counter sale. Although it may be purchased in pharmacies, supermarkets, and corner stores, it may not always be next to the Tylenol. Many stores keep naloxone locked up or behind the pharmacy counter, so you may have to ask a store clerk if they carry it. A recent study in Houston found that only 28 percent of the pharmacies that sold naloxone kept it on the shelves. Some insurance providers will cover naloxone for the simple price of a co-pay, but you must have a prescription. In Connecticut, pharmacists, who have undergone special training in naloxone, are allowed to write prescriptions for it. If you have insurance, ask them to write you a prescription so you will only have to pay a co-pay instead of the full price. There is no age limit on who can buy naloxone, and no ID is required. Naloxone can also be purchased directly from the manufacturer, online from the pharmacy, or even from some online retailers like Amazon. Public health departments and harm reduction services such as syringe exchange sites also provide free naloxone and training. A typical training for naloxone takes only a few minutes. In some parts of the country, naloxone is available in vending machines either for a small price or free. Some jurisdictions are now putting naloxone in public access boxes similar to those used for automatic defibrillators (AEDs) or in the same machine next to the AED.

HOW SHOULD NALOXONE BE STORED?

Naloxone should be protected from temperature extremes and direct sunlight.

DOES NALOXONE EXPIRE?

Technically naloxone does expire, but it should still work for years after its expiration date. Recently, the FDA extended the naloxone expiration date from three years to four years after previously extending it from two years to three. One study showed naloxone stayed viable even after 30 years of storage in a less-than-ideal setting. If someone is overdosing and your expired naloxone is all you have, use it.

CAN SOMEONE USE NALOXONE ON THEMSELVES?

Naloxone is indicated for depressed respirations in a patient unresponsive to stimulation. Once someone is in this state of overdose, they are in no position to self-administer naloxone. That said, there have been instances of people who self-administered naloxone after using opioids because they felt something amiss, as if they knew they were about to become unresponsive, and thereby prevented themselves from overdosing. I have had patients say something similar. They used opioids, suddenly felt strong effects, and quickly administered naloxone. People who use drugs, however, should not rely in any way on their ability to do this. Yet for people who use opioids alone, which is not recommended, it is not a bad practice to have naloxone at their side so that anyone who finds them will have quick access to the naloxone as well as a clue to the cause of their unresponsiveness.

Can I Get in Trouble for Giving Someone Naloxone (e.g., Good Samaritan Laws)?

Most states have Good Samaritan laws to protect people who assist an overdosed person in a good faith attempt to save them. In the Bible, a good Samaritan stops and aids a stranger injured by the side of the road after others have crossed the street to avoid the victim. While laws vary from state to state, many protect people from liability for causing injury as well as arrest for drug use and possession if they report an overdose. Laws will not protect people, however, if they are possessing drugs with the intent to sell them or if they have sold the drug to the person who overdosed. Additionally, if a mother overdoses in front of her children, a good Samaritan law will not protect her from a possible intervention from child services. States with Good Samaritan laws do have lower overdose death rates, according to the US Government Accountability Office.

NALOXONE MYTHS

Myth: Naloxone Requires Multiple Doses to Reverse Today's Stronger Opioids

Newer synthetic fentanyls do not require more doses of naloxone than traditional fentanyl to reverse an overdose. While the opposite has been speculated, including by manufacturers of high dose naloxone, studies have refuted this. In Connecticut, a review of EMS data from 2020 to 2023 showed there was no year-to-year increase in naloxone dosing. Eighty-four percent of patients responded to one full dose or less of naloxone, with the one full dose being either 2 mg or less by the IV or IM route or 4 mg or less by the intranasal route. EMS often gives small amounts of naloxone (less than a full dose) titrated to effect to help avoid precipitated withdrawal. Naloxone just needs to regain 50 percent of the receptors responsible for breathing to reverse an opioid overdose. To date, no opioid has been found not to respond to naloxone.

Regarding dosage, follow the naloxone administration instructions, monitor for breathing, and give an additional dose only if breathing is inadequate.

Myth: Naloxone Encourages Drug Use by Providing a Safety Net for Users

A 2019 economics paper entitled "The Moral Hazard of Lifesaving Innovations: Naloxone Access, Opioid Abuse, and Crime" argued that increasing access to naloxone permits risky behavior, unintentionally increases opioid use, leads to more crime, and may increase the death rate. The paper generated a great deal of controversy. The coauthors' underlying assumption is that naloxone creates a safety net that encourages opioid use because users know they can be revived if they overdose. The authors cite a legislator who, at a congressional hearing, said, "Kids are having opioid parties with no fear of overdose"; news reports of police finding naloxone at overdose scenes; and an Ohio police officer who said, "We've Narcan'd the same guy 20 times." The coauthors say their data prove that these anecdotes represent valid concerns, even if the Narcan party's anecdote seems to have little validity. Other research papers have come to the opposite conclusion. A paper published in the journal *Addictive Behaviors* shows a small decrease in heroin use among users who underwent naloxone training. A paper published in the journal *Addiction* that reviewed 22 naloxone studies found that naloxone training programs reduced overall mortality among those trained.

Myth: Patients Who Receive Naloxone Will Overdose Repeatedly in the Future, and Many Will Die Within a Year

Most overdoses are accidental. Users are not trying to overdose; they are only seeking either temporary euphoria, to feel normal due to their dependence, or to stop feeling sick from withdrawal. While there are documented reports of users overdosing multiple times, they are the exception. CDC data showed that in 2021, only 11.6 percent of fatal overdoses had a documented prior overdose in their records. In Connecticut, 16 percent of fatal overdose patients had a previously reported overdose within the last year. While the true number of repeat overdoses is likely higher due to cases where patients overdosed and 911 was not called, clearly not every patient who overdoses has a history of frequent overdose. A study in Western Pennsylvania found that 15 percent of patients who overdosed and were taken to the hospital had a repeat overdose within the year, and 3.5 percent of them died of overdose. Having an overdose requiring naloxone is a risk factor for future overdose or death, but it is not a guarantee.

Myth: Patients Who Receive Naloxone Are Always Violent After Resuscitation

Patients who have overdosed, particularly if they are put into withdrawal by naloxone, may be agitated. A user may be frustrated that they feel sick from the withdrawal, upset to be robbed of their high, upset over losing the money they just spent to purchase the drugs, and upset that the overdose occurred. In data from Connecticut, only 1 in 200 patients revived with naloxone required sedation from EMS crews to manage their combativeness. There were no reports of EMS crews being physically attacked by revived drug users in the period studied.

Mother

The woman watched the man's head fall back and his mouth open, but he didn't slip from his seat on the city bus. He began to snore. It was irregular and somewhat gasping, and then he was quiet. "I wish I could sleep like that," the man sitting across from her said. The woman wasn't the type to speak up, but she kept wondering if maybe the man wasn't just sleeping; maybe he had overdosed. They were on Park Street, where her daughter told her she came to buy drugs before she'd finally agreed to go to treatment. She was home now and doing well, but at her doctor's suggestion, the woman kept naloxone both at home and in her purse just in case. With her daughter foremost in her mind, she blurted it out. "I think he's overdosed," she said.

"He's just drunk," the man across from her said. "I wouldn't bother him."

She stood and approached the driver. "Ma'am, I think there is a passenger who is sick."

The driver pulled the bus to the side of the road and then walked back to the young man. She gave him a little push, but he did not respond. She swore under her breath, then walked back to the front of the bus, picked up her radio, and told her dispatcher they needed an ambulance. "I'm not allowed to do anything more than that," she said to the woman.

The other passengers shouted at the man to wake up. The woman shook his shoulder. His chest heaved, but then it was motionless. She reached forward and opened one of his eyelids. He didn't flinch. His pupils were pinpoint. She noticed the skin around his lips now had a bluish tint. She opened her purse and took out her naloxone. She had never used it before, but she followed the training they'd given her. She tore the blister pack open, removed the device, stuck the nozzle in the man's nose, and pushed the plunger. She waited for several moments and then gave him another shake.

The young man gasped. He still wasn't awake, but his chest was moving again.

"I think it's working," another rider said.

By the time my partner and I boarded the bus, the young man had opened his eyes. He was jittery and perspiring. The people on the bus were applauding. "What happened?" I asked the onlookers.

The woman, who was visibly trembling, said, "I gave him Narcan." She held up the vial she still held in her hand. "He wasn't breathing right, so I gave it to him."

"You did right, girl!" a woman sitting nearby said.

I nodded and then turned to the young man. "You're not in trouble, but we should probably take you to the hospital for evaluation."

"I just fell asleep," the young man said. "I just fell out."

I picked up the small torn glassine envelope that lay on the seat next to the man like it had fallen out of the pocket of his hoodie. I read the printed writing on it, right under the blue-and-black skull. "Stranger Danger."

The young man said nothing. He looked down at his hands.

"It's okay," I said. "We'll take you to the hospital. There will be someone you can talk with there about getting into treatment if that's something you're ready for."

A firefighter helped him up and led him outside to where my partner was now putting a clean sheet on the stretcher. I stayed for a moment and talked to the woman, who told me what happened and how she only carried the Narcan because of her daughter. Her voice broke with emotion as she talked.

"Good work," I said. "You did well."

That evening when she reached home, I imagined her finding her daughter studying in her room. She hugs her and makes no attempt to hide her tears.

CHAPTER 4

911 and Beyond

CALL 911

When you encounter a person who has overdosed, call 911 early. Get help on the way. When you call 911, your call is answered by an emergency dispatcher. Depending on where you live, the dispatcher could be in a large regional center with many operators, or they could be one person sitting alone in front of a console in a small police department. While the dispatcher asks you what your emergency is, your address should already be appearing on their screen. The dispatcher will ask you a series of questions, but don't worry about it delaying anything; responders should already be on the way. Again, depending on where you live, there will be different agency responses. In most systems, the first responders who arrive will be either police or fire. An ambulance crew should follow shortly after or may arrive first if they are in the area when the call goes out.

If you are at home, **make certain your house is well lit and marked so the responders know which house to enter.** While GPS has made it easier for EMS to find the correct

911 AND BEYOND

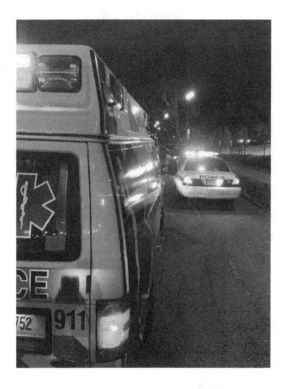

house, it is sometimes difficult to find the right one, particularly when houses are close together. This can be further complicated if neighbors turn on their lights and open their doors to see what is going on. I have many tales of going to the wrong doorway or running through the hallways of an apartment building trying to find the right apartment. If someone else is with you, have them stand by a door to flag the responders. If you are in an apartment, leave the door open, or if possible, send someone down to the lobby or front entrance to escort the responders to the right apartment by the quickest route.

FIRST RESPONDER ARRIVAL

First responders will begin assessing the patient while asking you what happened. Do your best to describe the state you found the patient in, how you recognized the overdose, what you did to treat it, and what you have seen posttreatment. Any information you have about what substances were used and the routes can all be helpful.

EMS CARE

Responders may administer additional naloxone if naloxone hasn't already been given or if it has been given and the patient continues to have depressed respirations. Responders will also position the patient to make certain their windpipe, or what we call the airway, is open and not blocked. If breathing is depressed, responders will use a bag-valve device, which consists of a plastic mask that they seal over the patient's nose and mouth and an attached balloon-type bag that they squeeze to send air into the patient's lungs. They may also insert a plastic device in the person's nose or mouth to keep the tongue from occluding the airway. Sometimes inserting this device or even pressing a mask against a patient's face stimulates them enough to rouse them. Administering oxygen itself can sometimes revive an overdose victim if their opioid load isn't too much. If the crew can effectively ventilate (move oxygen into the lungs and carbon dioxide out) a person with a bag-valve-mask, they could in theory continue to do so until the opioid wears off even without administering naloxone, but the time to resuscitation could be lengthy—hours in some cases—compared with naloxone's quick time to action.

Ambulance crews will usually stay on scene, deferring transport, until the naloxone has had a chance to work and the patient no longer needs bag-valve-mask ventilation. It is much easier to provide care on scene than while carrying a limp patient who needs to be ventilated down stairs and out to the ambulance.

EMS AND CARDIAC ARREST

Crews will also stay on scene if the patient is in cardiac arrest, meaning the patient's heart has stopped. The responders will provide CPR and administer the cardiac drug epinephrine through an IV or intraosseous (IO) line to try to restart the heart. Paramedic crews carry all the equipment and medications needed to resuscitate a patient in opioid overdose on scene. Their focus is on providing perfect cardiac compressions and effective ventilations to keep the brain perfused with oxygen-rich blood until the heart can be restarted. Naloxone is ineffective at this point. Remember, self-sustained breathing cannot be restored if the heart is not working.

CPR is usually ineffective when a patient is being moved. This is also true of attempting CPR in moving ambulances, where every bump or sudden turn can lead to hands coming off the chest and a disruption of the necessary cadence. If a patient in nontraumatic (not caused by a blunt or penetrating injury) cardiac arrest is not resuscitated on scene, there is little hope they will be successfully resuscitated at the hospital, except in certain rare circumstances. A person in traumatic cardiac arrest likely needs a surgeon and capabilities that an ambulance crew cannot typically provide. These patients receive a short scene time with rapid transport, known as "load and go." Even then their prognosis is grim. Few patients who are transported in any type of cardiac arrest survive in comparison to patients who are resuscitated on scene.

POST-RESUSCITATION ASSESSMENT

Most people who receive naloxone before their heart has stopped effectively beating do well. As mentioned, a person who is addicted to opioids may be sick or agitated after being resuscitated, particularly if given large amounts of naloxone. The naloxone has wiped the opioids out of their system, and the drug has put them into withdrawal. Their bodies, which have become dependent on opioids, are now suddenly without opioids and will react negatively.

Patients may be agitated after naloxone resuscitation, but they are rarely truly violent toward others. It is not uncommon for people to deny drug use, particularly if law enforcement responded to the call. In most jurisdictions today, law enforcement will not arrest people who have overdosed. Their concern is increasingly helping people find the treatment resources they need.

The EMS responders will evaluate a person post-resuscitation. EMS will reassess a patient's vital signs and check their oxygen saturation. Some people get stomach contents into their lungs when they overdose. This is known as aspiration. Aspiration may cause low oxygen saturation and coarse sounds in the lungs. In aspiration, the lungs are damaged and unable to take full advantage of the oxygen they are breathing in. It is important that post-resuscitation patients with low oxygen saturations be seen at the hospital for treatment. They may require supplemental oxygen as well as antibiotics and skilled care. Patients suffering from post-resuscitation pulmonary edema will also require skilled hospital care and monitoring. Pulmonary edema usually resolves in a day or two.

EMS will always recommend that patients who have suffered overdose go to the hospital for monitoring and further evaluation. Naloxone does not last as long as many opioids, so there is a concern that someone will relapse into an overdosed state. This is far more likely if the person ingested time-released pills than if they injected heroin or fentanyl. Most studies have shown very little risk of subsequent overdose from patients who receive naloxone and then refuse transport to the hospital.

If a person is alert and oriented post-overdose, they have a right to refuse transport to the hospital. If they do refuse transport, it is important that someone stays with them to make certain they don't re-overdose.

Many EMS services are now leaving naloxone kits with patients, their families, and their friends. The kits include not only naloxone and a face shield (if rescue breathing is needed) but also information on where to access help and other needed resources. Patients who do refuse may feel driven to use again, particularly if the naloxone puts them into withdrawal.

A few EMS services are now offering a dose of buprenorphine to naloxone-resuscitated patients in withdrawal. As we will discuss later in this chapter, buprenorphine is a type of opioid that does not produce euphoria but can help ameliorate opioid craving. To date, these programs are not widespread in the prehospital environment but are increasingly available in EDs.

HOSPITAL

The hospital provides further evaluation as well as an opportunity for intervention and treatment. For patients who have already been revived and are alert and breathing on their own, the hospital can monitor them for a few hours in a safe environment and ideally can help evaluate their health, including their mental health needs. They can then direct the patients to social services and treatment opportunities. Unfortunately, not all EDs have the resources to help people who have overdosed get the follow-up care they need. Services can be sparse.

Many people who use drugs feel that they are stigmatized by ED health care providers. They may be made to feel that they are taking up valuable ED time that could be spent treating more deserving patients. Their complaints may not be taken seriously, and their pain and withdrawal symptoms may be ignored or undertreated. After observing a patient for two hours, the hospital may discharge them with instructions to "STOP USING FENTANYL!" Patients may also be given a list of treatment programs that have lengthy waiting lists. These patients are then sent back out to the streets, even those who are in active drug withdrawal and are in danger of using again just to keep the sickness at bay. Fortunately, many hospitals are now changing their approach.

RECOVERY NAVIGATORS

Recovery navigators are people in long-term recovery who work at hospitals either as hospital staff or contracted from social service agencies. They meet with overdose patients in the ED and continue to work with them after they are discharged. The navigators talk them through the various recovery and treatment options to find one that might work for them. They try to take a whole-person mind, body and spirit approach that looks at all aspects of a person's situation, including a range of social service needs. Do they have food to eat or a safe place to live? Such an approach with a recovery navigator has shown that patients are more likely to engage in treatment.

BUPRENORPHINE THERAPY

Some hospitals offer buprenorphine, an FDA-approved treatment for opioid use disorder, in the ED to patients who are in drug withdrawal. Buprenorphine, also known as Suboxone, is a long-acting opioid that reduces withdrawal symptoms (e.g., body aches, nausea, vomiting, and diarrhea) as well as opioid cravings without providing the intense euphoria of heroin or fentanyl. Patients can get an induction dose in the ED and then are scheduled for follow-up care and treatment in an addiction clinic. If the patient is in withdrawal, the buprenorphine will ease the side effects and help prevent them from seeking additional illicit opioids to vanquish their sickness.

ED DISPOSITION

An ED may keep a patient overnight and then arrange to transport them directly to a treatment center the next day if there is an opening and the patient agrees to enter treatment. If the patient is being discharged, some hospitals will provide take-home naloxone. Other hospitals may routinely throw away a drug user's gear, including the clean syringes they may have obtained from a syringe services program. Some hospitals are now providing safe-use kits to users to ensure if they do use, they don't resort to sharing needles with others, which can spread diseases like HIV and hepatitis C. These kits are often provided to the hospitals by local harm reduction agencies.

HOSPITAL ADMISSION

Patients who cannot be resuscitated fully by EMS, who continue to have low oxygen saturations, or who have other identified medical problems may be admitted to the hospital or, if appropriate, the intensive care unit (ICU) for further care. While most patients recover their ability to breathe on their own within 2–15 minutes of receiving naloxone, if the person has been without oxygen for a longer period, their brains may have been stunned, and returning to consciousness may take longer. Hypothermia (excess cold) and hypercarbia (a buildup of carbon dioxide) may further delay mental response.

People who have suffered prolonged hypoxia often end up with anoxic brain injury, injury caused by prolonged lack of oxygen to the brain. The brain is damaged to a degree that it cannot recover to full functioning. A person's heart may be beating again, but the brain is no longer able to function to responsiveness. Anoxic brain injury is particularly a problem with patients whose hearts were stopped and needed prolonged resuscitation. Some of these patients will gradually recover in the coming days, but for others, brain scans may show that the damage sustained was both severe and permanent. Rather than live in a vegetative state, some patients are provided comfort measures only (CMO) after consultation with their families. They are given pain medicine and removed from the ventilators. Some donate their organs.

Mate

Welfare check. A visiting nurse came, but no one would answer the door. She could hear a radio playing. The superintendent lets us in. The apartment is a poor man's Hoarderville, with open boxes and dirty clothes stacked as high as the unwashed dishes in the sink. The man is sitting at a table with his head in his hands, a chessboard in front of him. For a moment, I fear he is not breathing, but when I nudge him, he moves. He turns slowly and stares blankly at me. I ask if he is okay, but he doesn't answer. I nudge him again, but he is out of it. I try to get him to squeeze my hands, but he doesn't follow any commands. Still, he has a decent pulse, and his breathing, while a bit slow, is even.

His medications are on the table alongside the chessboard. I read the labels. Metoprolol and HCTZ for hypertension, furosemide for congestive heart failure, simvastatin for high cholesterol, coumadin for atrial fibrillation and blood clots, allopurinol for gout, metformin for diabetes, oxycodone for pain, Colace to soften his stool. As I reach for each bottle, I can't help but admire the antique chessboard; the pieces are large and carved from wood. No idle purchase.

I always wonder about my patients' lives. On the wall is a picture of a strong man in military uniform and another with the same man surrounded by a large family. There are many pictures of younger children. The pictures are old and faded.

We pick him up, me with my hands under his arms and a firefighter grabbing his legs. It is then I see the torn heroin bag on the floor below the chair. I check his eyes once we have him strapped in on the stretcher. His pupils are pinpoint. Damn. It never ceases to amaze me how widespread heroin use is in the city. He is breathing well enough that I don't need to give him any naloxone. All he needs is a little shake to keep his breathing up when he nods off.

I wonder how many years he has been using and where he gets the heroin from. By the door is a walker, the kind with tennis balls on the ends to make for smoother rolling. Did he push his walker all the way down to Park Street to get his $3 bag, or does his dealer knock on the door with a regular delivery?

Was he once one of those who played chess in the park for a dollar a game? When was the last time he played a fellow human, relegated now to playing against himself in this dim apartment? I wonder if he replays lost games from his past, like many chess masters do, studying them to see where they went wrong. Maybe the heroin helps him play better, relaxing him and letting his mind see patterns that reveal the proper move.

I pick up my gear as we prepare to head down to the ambulance. I take a last look at the chessboard. I am new to the game, but it looks like if he is playing black, he is in a losing position. White's pawns are advancing on his king, and his two rooks are about to be forked by the opposing knight. Soon his pieces will join those already taken, standing helpless now on the sidelines among his battalion of prescription pill bottles. The battle will come to an end. As it will one day for us all.

PART TWO

Understanding the Crisis

CHAPTER 5

Fentanyl

The Present Danger

The first wave of the current opioid epidemic began in 1996 with the aggressive marketing of the prescription opioid painkiller OxyContin. The manufacturer, Purdue Pharma, targeted general practitioners and developed materials promoting the aggressive and escalating use of opioids for pain conditions while minimizing the addiction risk. The company stated that OxyContin had less than a 1 percent chance of addiction, that it could not produce a high, and that users could not build up a tolerance to it. It was a lie. None of the company's statements were true, and they knew it. Physicians gave too many pills for too many days at too strong a strength. As prescriptions rose, so did addiction, overdose, and death. In time, users learned to crush the time-released pills into powder and then snort or inject the drug to achieve the full high immediately.

The second wave of the epidemic began in 2010 when users switched to heroin after an abuse-resistant formula of

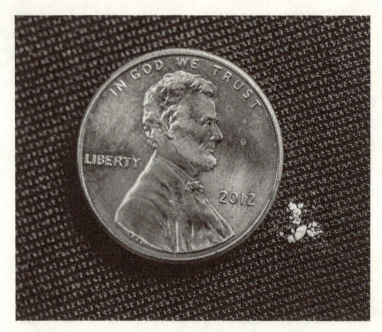

Lethal dose of fentanyl compared with a penny

OxyContin was introduced. The reformulated pills made it harder for users to crush the pills into usable powder. Heroin was cheaper, stronger, and more readily available. It has been estimated that 80 percent of people addicted to heroin first misused prescription drugs. The death rate skyrocketed.

The third and deadliest wave of the opioid epidemic began in 2013 when the heroin supply was increasingly adulterated with illegally produced fentanyl. Fentanyl, a synthetic opioid manufactured in laboratories, is 50 times stronger than heroin and 100 times stronger than morphine by weight. Fentanyl has a rapid onset and a short duration of action that has made it a widely used alternative to morphine for quick-acting pain relief. It is routinely used in surgery and is also used for palliative care in the form of a fentanyl patch specially engineered to be placed on the skin to deliver pain relief over an extended period. As a paramedic, I carry both morphine and fentanyl. I usually choose fentanyl for my patients because it acts much more rapidly and does not last as long as morphine. It is a great prehospital drug, providing immediate pain relief that lasts through transport and hospital intake. A doctor can then choose whether to continue pain medication. While fentanyl is 100 times stronger than morphine by weight, it is issued in vials of 100 micrograms (mcg), while morphine is issued in vials of 10 mg. This means a vial of 100 mcg of fentanyl is equivalent to 10 mg vial of morphine. Both versions are easy to dose and consistently provide appropriate relief.

The fentanyl killing people across our country is not medical-grade fentanyl stolen from hospital pharmacies or medical warehouses. The fentanyl sold on the street is illegally manufactured in clandestine labs and comes mainly in the form of a white powder that is hard to distinguish visually from white powdered heroin, making it easy for dealers to add it to heroin or sell it in place of heroin when combined with adulterants (e.g., sugar, baking powder, or other substances discreetly mixed with the advertised drug to add more volume). The key factor in increasing deaths is that fentanyl, because it is so much more potent than heroin by weight, is difficult for dealers to evenly distribute when mixing their batches with adulterants and filling small packages meant for street sale, or in pressing the powder into pill form. If poorly mixed, a single small package or pill can cause death.

Dealers first added a bit of fentanyl to increase the potency of their heroin, but in most parts of the country, fentanyl has gradually come to displace heroin almost entirely. The reason for this is not consumer driven. Users did not demand it. The change came from the dealers. Fentanyl is simply much more profitable for them than heroin. Heroin needs to be grown in fields. Its production is dependent on weather, pestilence, and avoiding police who might burn down the fields. Once harvested, the heroin has to be carried from the fields to the place where it is refined, packaged, and then smuggled across the border. Fentanyl is not reliant on weather conditions or the threat of insects. The dealers don't have to worry about drones flying overhead to spot their fields. The most important feature of fentanyl is its strength, which makes it much more easily trafficked. Fifty times as much can be smuggled in the same size container, or the same potency can be smuggled in a container fifty times smaller. Even if cut to only

10 percent strength by drug cartels, it is still higher potency in a smaller parcel. A kilo of heroin and a kilo of fentanyl might cost the same to produce, but a kilo of fentanyl will produce 50 times greater profit if priced at the same potency. If priced at double the potency (twice as strong as heroin), it is still making 25 times as much profit. It is this huge profit margin that is behind the fentanyl epidemic.

Fentanyl has other properties that make it better for the dealers and more dangerous for the users. One is the length of the high. Heroin typically lasts six to eight hours before someone who is addicted to it starts to feel sick. Fentanyl lasts three to four hours. Some users may require redosing even more frequently than these time intervals to avoid getting sick. If you are addicted to fentanyl, you will need to use it more often than someone who is addicted to heroin would need to use heroin. To help extend the high, users are increasingly using cocaine or methamphetamine to keep them energized while they find the money for their next buy. The bottom line is more sales for the dealers.

An additional factor benefiting the dealers is that fentanyl has high lipophilicity, which means it stores easily in the body's fat system. For people who use fentanyl regularly and are trying to quit, this means that the fentanyl that has accumulated over time in the body fat slowly ebbs out, making it harder for the body to clear itself entirely of fentanyl. This causes a stronger and more prolonged withdrawal.

Withdrawal is horribly painful, and many users can't endure the suffering knowing that they can cure the withdrawal agony simply by using again. Fentanyl is thus more addictive than heroin and harder to kick.

Fentanyl's potency has other devastating effects. Today, anyone can order fentanyl on the dark web and have it delivered to their home by mail or a shipping carrier. This means the bar for becoming a dealer is very low. No more driving to the wrong side of town to meet a man who knows a man who has two bodyguards who might kill you just because they don't like the way you look at their boss. A single, 1 oz envelope of pure fentanyl from China contains enough active ingredient that, when combined with adulterants, can make 28,000 doses at 1 mg of fentanyl per dose—more than enough to start a small-scale drug empire.

THE CUTTING PROCESS: NOT A SCIENCE

Both heroin and fentanyl are cut (adulterated) with substances like sugar, baking soda, and other white-colored powders. Adulterating the drug produces more product to sell and helps ensure that the product is not too potent. Typically, heroin is cut or adulterated to perhaps 50 percent heroin, 50 percent adulterant. Fentanyl should be cut to 1 percent active ingredient, 99 percent adulterant if sold in a 0.1 g package. That's easy to do if you are a multibillion-dollar pharmaceutical company with top scientists and labs with the latest state-of-the art equipment, but not so easy if you are a street-level drug dealer doing the mixing on your kitchen table using a blender made for protein shakes. Whether you received your fentanyl pure from China or cut to 10 percent potency from Mexico, getting a consistent 1 mg dose in every 0.1 g $3 bag you package is difficult. Fentanyl tends to clump, which can create the chocolate chip cookie effect. One bag might contain a giant clump (chip) of fentanyl, while another bag might not have any chips. A 0.1 g bag of cut "fentanyl" contains 100 mg of powder by weight. Just 2 mgs of fentanyl are considered a potentially lethal dose by the Drug Enforcement Administration (DEA). How do you safely measure the correct dose at the kitchen table so that each bag you fill with a tiny spoon has only 1 percent fentanyl?

UNSAFE SUPPLY

The number one reason people are dying today of fentanyl overdose is that users cannot judge their dose. Even if you are the most experienced user, there is no way for you to tell that the white powder you poured into your cooker (a bottle-cap-sized container), mixed with saline, and then drew up with your syringe and are now pushing into your vein is 1 percent fentanyl or 10 percent fentanyl—the latter being a dose that will kill you if you are using alone and no one finds you before your heart stops beating five minutes after the fentanyl has stopped your breath cold.

OVERDOSE EPIDEMIC OR POISONING EPIDEMIC?

The term *overdose epidemic* has become a misnomer. It is a poisoning epidemic. Imagine if you drank a glass of wine in a bar, and that wine was 100 percent alcohol instead of 12 percent alcohol as labeled, but you couldn't taste the difference. A couple of glasses could kill you by alcohol poisoning. If it was determined the bottle of wine you drank from was incorrectly labeled, the government would institute an immediate recall to protect others from being poisoned. In 1982 when seven people died from cyanide-contaminated Tylenol bottles that had been tampered with, Johnson & Johnson recalled 31 million bottles of the over-the-counter pain reliever. Protecting the public came before profits. Unfortunately, there are no consumer protections for illicit drug users. Outside of legalization and government regulation of a safe supply, which I don't think America is ready for politically, the government has no mechanism to recall illicit fentanyl even though it is causing sudden poisoning deaths in tens of thousands of Americans.

The poisoning versus overdose labeling is a controversial topic. *Overdose* implies a person took too many doses. It also implies the person who died was a "drug addict" and the fault was theirs for taking too much of a substance. *Poisoning* implies that the victim had no intention of killing themselves or even getting high. They may have merely been trying to ease their back pain by taking a Percocet given to them by a friend. Maybe they were just taking what they thought was enough to make their withdrawal symptoms go away. It wasn't like they went to a bar and drank beer after beer until, sloppily drunk, they passed out. They had one dose (one beer), and they died. They were poisoned.

The problem with the word *poisoning*, some may argue, is that it implies a crime. Who poisoned the victim? Some law enforcement people have used this as a reason to prosecute the drug dealer, even if that "dealer" is a friend with substance use disorder who bought the drugs to share with the victim. Because he provided the drugs to the victim, he is responsible for the death. Or so goes the reasoning. I will talk about this more in chapter 10. After considering the argument, I stick with "poisoning" instead of "overdose." The people who are dying don't wish to die. They die because fentanyl cannot be safely mixed outside of a pharmaceutical company. We have fentanyl today because prohibiting substances inevitably leads to stronger, deadlier drugs. More on this in a later chapter.

FENTANYL TEST STRIPS

There are test strips that people can use to see if fentanyl is present in their powder. They do this by putting a little bit of water in the wax fold (the envelope fentanyl is sold in in some parts of the country) or in the cooker. They dip the test strip in the water and wait a minute to see if a red line appears in the appropriate spot. If the red line appears, fentanyl is confirmed, but it doesn't tell the crucial information—how much fentanyl is present.

DEATH NUMBERS

In Connecticut in 2012, 14 deaths were attributable to fentanyl (5 percent of all opioid deaths). By 2021, 1,312 people died of fentanyl poisoning, which represented 93 percent of all opioid deaths. In 2017, 90 percent of all heroin bags tested in Hartford, Connecticut, by local harm reduction workers contained fentanyl. In 2022, less than 10 percent of fatal opioid cases in the state tested positive for heroin.

According to the CDC, 88 percent of all US opioid deaths in 2021 involved fentanyl, and only 13 percent involved heroin. As mentioned, fentanyl started its reign of terror on the East Coast, where powdered heroin was prominent. Most heroin users west of the Mississippi generally used black tar heroin, a sticky, tarlike substance that has not been fully purified. Black tar heroin is typically smoked, but it can also be injected. The economics of fentanyl, however, have spread both fentanyl and the related deaths westward. Much of the fentanyl in the west is in the form of pressed pills.

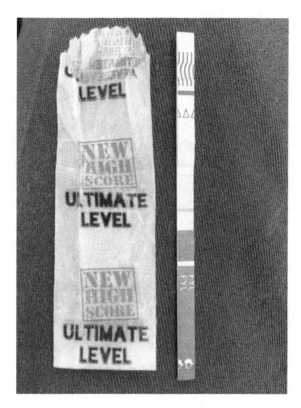

Fentanyl test strip (positive)

COUNTERFEIT PILLS

Years ago, if someone was worried that fentanyl might be in their heroin, they could seek safety in reverting to pharmaceutical pills like Percocet. Because Percocet came from a pharmaceutical company, people could be certain that all pills had the same advertised strength. Not anymore. Dealers are buying pill presses and dyes for Percocet 30s and other common opioid pills, then pressing powder and fentanyl into counterfeit pills that look just like the originals. In 2018, law enforcement seized 290,394 counterfeit pills containing fentanyl. In 2021, they seized 9,649,551. In 2023, the number was over 79 million. Users cannot easily tell an illegitimate counterfeit pill from an authentic pharmaceutical-grade pill. And like the fentanyl in the heroin bags, there is no way for a user to tell how much fentanyl is in the pill they just bought, even if they know it is a counterfeit pill. Is it 1 percent or 12 percent? An expected high or death? A 30 mg oxycodone pill weighs 135 mg. The pharmaceutically produced pill is composed of 30 mg of the active ingredient (22 percent by weight), but a fake oxycodone pill with just 2 percent fentanyl as the active ingredient (2.7 mg) would be considered lethal. Do you trust the dealer pressing the pills to put the exact same amount of fentanyl in each pill at a dose that is not lethal? In 2023, the DEA found that seven out of ten fake pills tested in their lab contained a potentially lethal dose, up from four out of ten in 2021.

It has been speculated that drug cartels are mass-producing counterfeit prescription pills to attract new users who may be averse to street fentanyl. Recently in Mexican border towns, American tourists have bought packaged pills in pharmacies sold as oxycodone that turned out to be counterfeit pills containing fentanyl. To date, no fake pills containing fentanyl have been found for sale in American pharmacies, where there are stronger safeguards.

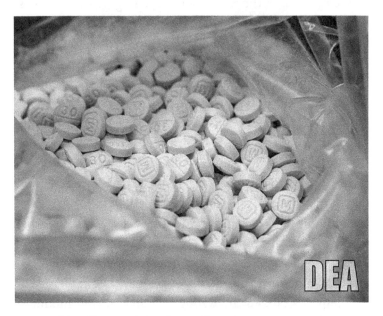

Counterfeit pills containing fentanyl

FENTANYL-CONTAMINATED COCAINE?

People who use cocaine are not safe from fentanyl, either. It is not uncommon to read newspaper headlines or hear on TV of multiple people who thought they were using cocaine to stop breathing moments after snorting their white powder. There has been wide speculation about whether dealers are intentionally lacing the cocaine to addict people, but I don't subscribe to that. Cocaine is addictive enough, plus I don't believe dealers want the reputation for selling tainted supplies. A more likely scenario is that the dealers who also sell fentanyl don't properly separate their two operations and don't use industrial techniques to sterilize their equipment. The same blender that was used to mix fentanyl is often used to mix cocaine. The same grainy wooden table is used to package the product. It takes just a small amount of fentanyl to get into cocaine to cause overdose and death.

My friend Kelley and her husband, Tom, worked for a dealer. In return for receiving a room to live in, each night they helped the dealer package his products. I asked her about the possibility of cocaine and fentanyl being mixed as her dealer sold both products. "Absolutely not," she said. "We have safeguards. We use different foil pans to do our mixing—one for fentanyl and one for cocaine. The other night, one of our helpers grabbed the wrong pan and started mixing. I spotted it and yelled at him. We have a reputation to uphold."

For all their good intentions, however, their safety standards are not government grade.

Stephen Murray, a former paramedic and overdose survivor and now full-time harm reductionist, made a remarkable video to demonstrate how easy it is for cross contamination to occur. He spread the spice turmeric (a red powder) on a wood table, cut it into lines, and then removed it. He then added salt to the apparently empty tabletop and began cutting it into lines. The white salt easily picked up splotches of the red turmeric that had hidden in the grains of the table. Had the turmeric been fentanyl and the salt cocaine, the resulting batch not only would have been contaminated, but it also would have been lethal to an opioid-naïve cocaine user.

FENTANYL-CONTAMINATED MARIJUANA?

There have been scattered reports in the media, including an anecdote in the *New York Times*, of fentanyl-contaminated marijuana. In Connecticut in 2021, police seized a marijuana sample from an overdose scene where a patient's overdose had been reversed with naloxone and sent it to the state forensic laboratory, where it tested positive for fentanyl. This combined with reports to the Connecticut Poison Control Center of patients overdosing after only smoking marijuana caused the state to issue an advisory. Further investigation, however, determined that the marijuana sample had been stored in the same container that had been used for fentanyl. Additionally, an investigation of the marijuana-only reports revealed many of the patients also had opioid histories. While these reports continue to come in occasionally, it is important to understand that they coincided with the legalization of marijuana in Connecticut and that many patients who are resuscitated with naloxone either claim they did not use drugs at all or deny the use of opioids. I had a patient once who said he had only smoked marijuana that he suspected was laced, but when we showed him the heroin bags we found on scene, he admitted he had used opioids. Some evidence suggests that fentanyl is an ineffective drug when smoked directly as its burn point is low enough that the user would be unable to get high if they smoked it in a joint. This is different from smoking fentanyl the traditional way by heating it up on foil and inhaling the vapors. If any dealers are lacing their marijuana with fentanyl, it is likely rare, done only by street-level dealers and not at the wholesale level, and it is most likely ineffective in providing a high or causing an opioid overdose.

CARFENTANIL

Carfentanil is another synthetic opioid used primarily to tranquilize large animals, such as elephants. It is purportedly 100 times stronger than fentanyl. It was attributed to a rise in deaths in several states, including Ohio and Pennsylvania, around 2017 before declining. In 2022, according to the CDC database, it was detected in only 6 of 18 reporting states and accounted for just 7 deaths, down from 28 deaths in 15 reporting states in 2021. The decline has been attributed to increased regulation of sources in China, but others believe the potency of the drug made it too hard to successfully blend into the drug supply without killing too many people. Unfortunately carfentanil deaths are upticking again with 168 deaths in 23 reporting state in 2023, although the number of cases is still small.

NITAZINES

Nitazines are novel synthetic opioids (NVOs) more powerful than fentanyl that have occasionally been detected in the US drug supply. Nitazines, like all opioids, respond to naloxone, despite speculation that they may require more naloxone than usual. Nitazines cannot be identified by fentanyl test strips. To date, nitazines have not been a strong presence on American streets. They accounted for 100 deaths in 2022 in 16 of 29 reporting states, down from 196 the previous year in 21 of 33 reporting states. The worry is that by clamping down on fentanyl, chemical manufacturers in China are going to continue to make ever-changing and stronger opioids with continually modified chemical structures to evade existing prohibitions. On the other hand, if they make the drugs too strong, the drugs will be far too risky for dealers to mix in a usable way.

XYLAZINE

Increasingly in the northeast and expanding across the country (found in 27 of 29 reporting states), a drug called xylazine is being added to fentanyl mixtures. Xylazine is an animal tranquilizer originally designed as an analgesic for people, but it was abandoned due to tests that showed it caused severe hypotension and depressed mental status. It is not an opioid and is not currently regulated. Drug dealers (likely at the local level) buy it and add it to their heroin-fentanyl mixture. Because fentanyl's high ebbs at three to four hours or sooner, adding xylazine adds "legs" to the drug, meaning the person's high lasts longer. Some users like this, but many don't. They can feel more stuporous and are slow to move. They are prone to blacking out, and the sedation can last much longer than sedation caused by fentanyl. The blackout effect poses an added risk for physical and sexual assault as well as injury from a fall due to suddenly passing out or blacking out for an extended period in a position that impedes blood flow to a limb. The concoction was first noticed in Puerto Rico in the early 2000s and later found a strong foothold in Philadelphia, where it is sold as "tranq dope." Here in Connecticut, it seems to just be used as an additive to fentanyl and is not typically requested or advertised, at least not by the users I have talked to. The real danger with xylazine is that it can cause severe skin necrosis, not only when injected but also when snorted or smoked. This is attributed to how it reduces oxygen uptake in the skin. Because xylazine is an analgesic, users often inject right back into the painful ulceration to provide temporary relief, which only makes the ulceration worse. There is also concern that withdrawal from xylazine is more difficult than withdrawal from fentanyl, so those who have been exposed to xylazine through their fentanyl mix may be less successful at completing detox and treatment.

There is debate as to whether xylazine is responsible for an increasing number of overdose deaths. A study on rats found that xylazine alone can lead to "sedation, muscle relaxation, decreased body temperature," and a "modest decrease in brain oxygen levels," but not nearly to the degree of heroin or fentanyl. The researchers found that when combined with heroin or fentanyl, xylazine caused oxygen levels to stay lower longer than with just fentanyl or heroin alone. This would suggest that it may lead to increased death. Anything that increases sedation may make someone already on the verge of respiratory arrest more likely to stop breathing and should be considered dangerous.

The biggest question: Is xylazine being added to fentanyl to enhance the product or used as a partial replacement for fentanyl? Clearly fentanyl is by far the more toxic drug. If xylazine, which is much cheaper than fentanyl ($6–$20 per kg versus $35,000–$50,000 per kg for fentanyl, according to the DEA), is added to the mix and consequently less fentanyl is used, the result could be fewer deaths and overdoses. A multicenter study involving nine EDs from 2020 to 2021 found that overdose victims who had both fentanyl and xylazine in their system were less likely to die than those who had fentanyl alone. They speculated that this was because those with xylazine likely had less exposure to fentanyl than those who tested positive only for fentanyl. Additionally, because xylazine helps extend the sedation of fentanyl, users use less often and thus have fewer chances to overdose. According to the Connecticut Office of the Chief Medical Examiner, xylazine was found in 24 percent of all of the state's fatal overdoses in 2022—roughly the same proportion of xylazine in the drug supply according to local testing. While the presence of xylazine rose 16.6 percent in fatal overdoses in 2022, fatal overdoses involving xylazine decreased by 4.7 percent.

Myth: Xylazine Is a Flesh-Eating Drug That Turns People into Zombies

"Xylazine, A Deadly Skin-Rotting Zombie Drug, Often Mixed w Fentanyl, Is on the Doorstep . . . Already Fueling a Horrific

Wave of Overdoses." This is the headline from a press release of US Senator Charles Schumer, a press release in which he promises to "supercharge" funding for law enforcement and interdiction to battle the xylazine threat. America has a history of hysteria over the drug war. From the era of *Reefer Madness* (a 1936 movie that showed how marijuana purportedly turned people into crazed villains) to the present day, the country has used fear to spark crackdowns against people who use drugs, to fund law enforcement, and to fuel political grandstanding to win votes. Xylazine does cause stupor, can lead to blackouts, and produces serious wounds, but it does not turn people into zombies, nor does it spread a flesh-eating disease. This characterization not only stigmatizes people who use drugs, but it has also been used to create hysteria and spur more funding for law enforcement.

FENTANYL MYTHS

There are several myths and widespread misinformation about fentanyl that need to be addressed because hysteria and false information stigmatize users and may prevent people from assisting overdose victims.

Myth: Touching Fentanyl Can Kill You

Headlines appear about law enforcement officers rushed to the hospital after being exposed to fentanyl. They were on scene when they encountered piles of powder, some of which got on their skin or was puffed into the air. They felt faint, and some even passed out. What happened? Did their exposure to fentanyl cause them to overdose? No. There is no danger of merely being exposed to fentanyl. For fentanyl to harm you, you have to inject it, snort it, or ingest it in significant quantities. It is not absorbed through the skin by casual contact. The skin is an effective barrier to powdered fentanyl. In fact, there are fentanyl dermal pads that are specially manufactured with a gel to enable absorption of the drug through the skin. It can take up to 12 hours for enough fentanyl to absorb through the skin to feel its analgesic effects.

So what causes the exposed law enforcement officers to pass out? The *nocebo effect*. The placebo effect is when someone feels better after taking a pill because they believe it is going to be good for them. The nocebo effect is when a person feels bad after taking a pill because they believe it is going to be bad for them. None of these police officers who are rushed to the hospital for fentanyl exposure ever test positive for fentanyl. The officers' signs and symptoms are not consistent with opioid overdose. Their typical complaints involve fainting, rapid heartbeats, and nausea, all more indicative of an anxiety attack than an opioid overdose. The root cause stems from a 2016 DEA announcement telling police officers that just touching fentanyl can be fatal. So unless that false information has been corrected, they think they are going to die when they are exposed to fentanyl. On July 27, 2017, the

American College of Medical Toxicology and the American Academy of Clinical Toxicology had to issue a joint statement, "Preventing Occupational Fentanyl and Fentanyl Analog Exposure to Emergency Responders," clarifying that "the risk of clinically significant exposure to emergency responders is extremely low." Eventually the DEA corrected their information, instructing those exposed to simply wash their hands with soap, but the rumor persists.

Myth: There Is Enough Fentanyl to Kill Everyone in the Country

Stories appear with regularity about the seizures of enough fentanyl to kill everyone in America. Again, this is hysteria. I could say there is enough water in the town lake to drown everyone in America, or enough bullets in the local gun store to kill everyone in the state. For the amount of fentanyl seized to kill everyone in America, everyone in America would have to roll up their sleeves, apply a tourniquet, and then consent to having someone push the syringe plunger into one of their arm veins. If you dropped the reported amount of fentanyl seized from an airplane and bombed Main Street with it, the only ones who would overdose are those who could find a big enough pile on the ground, stick their fingers in it, and then stick their powder-crusted fingers up their noses and forcibly inhale. The sad effect of these overblown headlines is to create fear that only further stigmatizes those who use drugs, which may prevent people from giving them needed aid for fear of suffering harm by having physical contact with them.

Myth: Rainbow Fentanyl Is Targeted to Children

Recently, law enforcement seized large amounts of multicolored counterfeit Percocet pills that contained fentanyl and were wrapped in Skittles packaging to conceal them from police. The DEA issued a warning that drug cartels were now targeting young Americans by making the drugs look like candy. News stories appeared across the country expressing concern that drug dealers were targeting children on Halloween to addict them and grow their customer base. You can be sure that on trick-or-treat night, dealers did not hand out $20,000 bags of "rainbow fentanyl" disguised as Skittles to 10-year-olds. Sometimes dealers hide drugs in fish, but when the drugs are discovered, no one writes news stories about drug dealers targeting cod lovers. Drugs and kids make for headlines, even when there is nothing to back them up. The real danger to kids is when those ages two and under are crawling around in houses where drugs are packaged or used openly. If they get into loose white powder and stick their fingers in their noses and inhale, then there may be a problem. Recently in the Bronx borough of New York, headlines surfaced when a one-year-old at a day care center died of an apparent fentanyl overdose. The day care center was used as a stash house for a local drug dealer. While not all these cases make headlines, they are not unheard of. In Connecticut between 2020 and 2022, there were 20 reports of youth two years and younger overdosing on opioids. The location of these calls included residences, a homeless shelter, a motor vehicle, and a bodega. EMS was able to recognize the opioid poisoning in most of the cases, but in others, they treated the children as unknown unresponsive or respiratory arrest, and it was only later in the hospital that the overdoses were uncovered after the children were given naloxone as a rule-out and responded to it.

FOURTH WAVE

Some have argued that there is a fourth wave of the opioid epidemic that includes the increasing use of fentanyl in combination with stimulants. Historically, epidemics of sedatives are followed by epidemics of stimulants. There has been a documented increase in the use of cocaine and methamphetamine and overall polysubstance use. Nationwide, 32.3 percent of fatal fentanyl overdoses involved stimulants. That only means that in 32.3 percent of the fatal overdoses, the person tested positive for both fentanyl and a stimulant, not necessarily that the stimulant was the cause of the patient's death. Here in Connecticut, the percentage of fatal fentanyl overdose victims who also tested positive for cocaine (the stimulant of choice in the area) rose from 22 percent in 2014 to 48 percent in 2022, steadily increasing every year except 2020. Speculation is that the short-acting fentanyl drives users to need stimulants to keep, extend, and heighten their high; decrease the risk of overdosing due to excess sedation; and give themselves enough energy to get enough money together to get their next fix. Stimulants, while decreasing the dangers of sedation, increase the risk for cardiovascular events such as heart arrhythmias, which can be lethal. Whether the presence of stimulants helps prevent overdose or worsens an overdose is based on each case. Regardless, the overdose death rate is still being driven by fentanyl.

Mascot

An emaciated man sits on a decrepit couch in the basement darkness; his right leg is folded up on his left knee as he probes his ankle for a vein. There is blood drawn back in the barrel. The small basement area is dirty; nearly a dozen used syringes lay on the table, along with torn heroin bags. In the corner in a broken laundry basket is a giant dust-encrusted bird head—the top half of a sports mascot outfit worn long ago.

The woman, who lives upstairs, heard him come in last night and then found him unresponsive this morning. She administered two vials of naloxone, which now lay on the cement floor, and then she called us. The man is cold to the touch and stiff—rigored into position, the needle still in his ankle, his lifeless hand still holding the syringe.

CHAPTER 6

Why People Use Drugs and the Science of Addiction

People have used opioids since the beginning of civilization. In the third millennium BC, the ancient Sumerians who lived in what is now Iraq cultivated the poppy seed and learned how to use opium derived from the seeds. They called it "the joy plant."

In Homer's *The Odyssey*, the Greek hero Odysseus and his men—worn out from the ten-year Trojan War, filled with sadness for the loss of their comrades, and beaten down by their long and difficult journey homeward—come to the island of the Lotus Eaters, where the inhabitants offer them a special plant to eat to ease their sorrow. Eating the lotus enables Odysseus's men to forget their heartaches. In "Lotos-Eaters," a poem by Alfred Lord Tennyson about the same tale, the Greek men beg the world to "let us alone" and welcome the lotus's power to make them forget. "Give us long rest or death, or dreamful ease," they beg. In one of the first interventions recorded in literature, Odysseus drags them back to the boats and restrains them; then those of his men who avoided the drug row fast, making their escape.

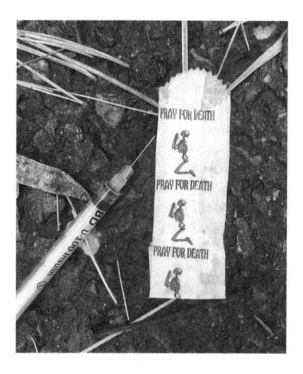

Unfortunately, the lotus of myth has never been limited to a distant island; it is all around us, in every community, and its power has only grown. Opium was used not only by the ancient Greeks but in later years by the Romans, Indians, the Chinese, and Europeans too. In 1806, morphine, named after Morpheus, the Greek god of sleep, was isolated from the opium plant. The American Civil War saw widespread use of morphine and the resulting addiction. In 1896, heroin was synthesized from the opium plant. Bayer, the company that later made aspirin, marketed heroin as a pain reliever, claiming it was not as addictive as morphine. Heroin was sold over the counter in drugstores. By 1924, prohibitionists had outlawed the drug due to its propensity to cause addiction. Soon thereafter, organized crime, recognizing a market for heroin, began to traffic in the drug. Heroin and now its successor, fentanyl, remain high-profit sources for organized criminals and drug cartels. Stiff criminal penalties have never deterred the drug trade, and cartels and dealers continue to flourish as the demand for opioids remains strong and there are profits to be made. While the legal threat may deter some, it clearly has not stopped the millions who struggle with substance use and those who use recreationally.

Societies outlaw drugs in the hopes that citizens will avoid health risks to themselves and the negative consequences of using drugs, which can lead to drug users breaking social contracts with their families, employers, and communities. This was why prohibition against alcohol was once the law of the land in our country. That prohibition was eventually overturned because it led to thousands of Americans being poisoned by illicit alcohol all while liquor use remained rampant despite its illegality. A similar situation exists with drugs today. The negative costs of prohibition are outweighing the intended consequences.

In a YouTube video, Dr. Gabor Maté, the author of the landmark book *In the Realm of Hungry Ghosts: Close Encoun-*

ters with Addiction, has a conversation with Guy Felicella, a former user of drugs and champion harm reduction advocate. Maté asks Felicella what the drugs did for him when he was struggling. He summarizes Felicella's response: "So the drugs gave you comfort, they gave you a sense of friendly acceptance, and they helped soothe your suffering. . . . Those are wonderful things. In other words, the drugs weren't your problem. Your drugs were an attempt to solve your problem." He goes on to say that while drugs can cause problems, they are not the primary problem. We need to address the primary problem, the roots of the sufferings that drive people to seek relief in drugs.

People don't use drugs to become lawbreakers, to disrupt their families or communities, or to threaten their own lives. People use drugs because the drugs work for what they need them to do, and that need can become so great it overrules everything else.

Austin Eubanks was a student at Columbine High School when two classmates shot him and killed his best friend along with so many others. He was prescribed painkillers for his injuries but found the pills worked best to blunt his emotional trauma. They helped him survive his great anguish. This boy who had never even smoked marijuana soon became addicted to heroin, alcohol, and methamphetamine. He fought addiction for over a decade before recovering and becoming a national speaker on drug use, offering his message of recovery and hope. I heard him speak in Hartford. Three weeks later he died of a drug overdose. Was it the drugs that killed him or the trauma he suffered that day in Columbine?

Not everyone who uses opioids becomes addicted. Some use only sporadically and can start and stop at will. Unfortunately for many, initial drug use does lead to addiction, based on their genes and environmental factors. Even for those who beat it, relapse is always a possibility, as it was for Austin Eubanks.

THE SCIENCE OF ADDICTION

The American Psychiatric Association defines addiction as "a complex condition, a brain disease that is manifested by compulsive substance use despite harmful consequence." The American Society of Addiction Medicine says addiction "is characterized by [an] inability to consistently abstain, impairment in behavioral control, craving, diminished recognition of significant problems with one's behaviors and interpersonal relationships, and a dysfunctional emotional response."

Opioids, which are among the most addictive substances, initially produce euphoria, an overwhelming response of dopamine in the brain, followed by an awareness of an ebbing of the drug and then for some, a preoccupation with reproducing the feeling. In time, some people's brains can become hijacked so people can no longer act in their best interest. These changes are so profound the damage can often be measured in images of the brain in the same way medical imaging can detect damaged hearts and lungs.

An analogy I have heard many substance use experts describe is one about fireworks. If you like pizza, imagine a firework of pleasure going off in your brain whenever you eat a slice. This is the neurotransmitter dopamine making you feel good about pizza. Sometimes, just thinking about pizza sets off a firework of pleasure. Now imagine you do heroin for the first time, and, particularly if you are genetically susceptible, instead of one firework going off in your brain, a Fourth of July grand finale of fireworks goes off in your brain. Your brain gets flooded with more dopamine than you have ever experienced before. The comedian Lenny Bruce described doing heroin as being like kissing God. Amazing, right? This explosion occurs in the part of the brain known as the basal ganglia, the pleasure center.

After a while, another part of the brain starts to notice the pleasure fading. This part of the brain is the extended amygdala, which sets off alerts about the withdrawal of the pleasure and causes anxiety. A third center, the prefrontal cortex, starts thinking about how you are going to get some more. In time, the fireworks set off in the pleasure center increasingly decrease, while the other centers go into overdrive: Help, I need more! I have to get more! The circuitry in the brain gets rewired. It becomes hijacked. The things that used to produce pleasure (dopamine)—such as eating, having sex, and taking care of children—no longer do. They can't compete with heroin, and the brain starts to believe heroin, which produces much higher levels of dopamine, is the key to the human's survival. The brain no longer processes information the way it once did. That's why people steal in front of security guards or shoot up drugs with their kids still in the car. That's why they use drugs when they know the drugs can kill them. To expect someone damaged by addiction to act rationally is akin to expecting someone with a broken leg to run the 100-yard dash or someone with heart and lung disease to climb Mount Everest in a storm.

People who are addicted see drugs in the same way they see the need to breathe and for their heart to beat. Drugs become central to their existence. Maslow's hierarchy of needs is a psychological theory consisting of five human needs, ranging from the basic physiological needs of breathing, eating, shelter, sleep, and reproduction to the highest levels of self-actualization and the desire to become the best one can be. For people addicted to drugs, getting and obtaining more drugs occupies that same basic layer of physiological need that comes before any of the other layers, including those of safety, love, esteem, and self-actualization.

Today scientists believe addiction is a chronic, relapsing brain disease that is caused by a confluence of factors, from genetics to environment and mental health. It cannot be cured acutely but needs long-term monitoring. Relapse is common. Even someone who has not used opioids for years can be triggered to use again. Addiction is not a character flaw.

OBJECTING TO THE BRAIN DISEASE STORY

I have met several people who use drugs who object to being characterized as having a brain disease. Not everyone who uses drugs has opioid use disorder, just as not everyone who drinks alcohol is an alcoholic. They may use drugs for other reasons but believe they are capable of stopping. That may be true for some people, but it clearly is not true for others. If we want to end drug-related deaths, those caught in addiction's web need help getting into treatment. Those who use drugs and are not addicted still need protection from our toxic street drug supply. I will discuss both treatment and harm reduction in future chapters.

Emerald City

She took the Dilaudid pill a friend offered her 12 years ago when she was 16. Her sister had recently died, and her young life, filled with depression and anxiety, had lost its only source of light. The pill made her feel well in a way she had never felt before. She liked who she was when she was on opioids. She had friends. She felt joy again. Four years later she tried heroin for the first time because it was cheaper and more accessible. Two years later she graduated to injecting. She's been to rehab five times with no success. She's tried methadone and Suboxone. No luck. She is on Vivitrol now, but as the monthly shot wanes, she always finds her way back to the nearby city. She injects herself with heroin because it soothes her anxiety and cushions her in a cloud of calm. She injects cocaine because it makes her feel invincible.

The guy she was with in the hotel room called 911 when he came out of the bathroom and found her unresponsive on the carpet with the two syringes on the bureau, the torn heroin bags branded "Emerald City," and the small plastic bag with some cocaine powder still in it.

She was blue with agonal respirations and vomit on the rug next to her. With some stimulation, bagging, and a small, titrated amount of naloxone, we brought her around. She didn't want to go to the hospital at first, but we convinced her she needed to be evaluated. Her heart was racing in the 140s, and her oxygen saturation was only in the high 80s. We were concerned she may have aspirated.

The now-silent man fetched her purse and slippers, and we put them on the back of the stretcher. With a blanket I covered her tattooed back and shoulders, but not before complimenting her on her artwork. The artist had drawn a magnificent mountaintop with elaborate etchings of trees, eagles, deer, and stars, along with the words "The journey to the top is my soul."

This is the third time she has overdosed but the first in three years. I give her my harm reduction talk about the dangers of fentanyl, how it mixes poorly so you never know how much you are actually getting in each $3 bag—none, a regular dose, or a lethal one. It was good she was not alone.

We talk more. She answers my question about how she got started, and she tells why it is so hard to quit. When I ask her who the man in the room was, she just shrugs. Some guy. I get her demographics. She lives in a small town 40 minutes from the city. She asks if she has to give me her emergency contact.

"No," I say. "Not if you don't want to give it."

"I don't want my parents to know."

"They don't have to. It's your choice."

"I don't want them to lose faith in me."

I ask her about her relationship with them, and she begins crying. "They love me," she says.

She tells me how supportive of her they have been, how much they care for her and want her to win her battle.

At the hospital, I tell the girl's story to the nurse, but the nurse just rolls her eyes. It is busy in the ED, and she has no time beyond a basic report.

I wonder where the girl is tonight. Is she home with her parents? What will they think when she asks to go out? Will she just walk the quiet small-town streets, struggling for the strength to stay the sober course, to keep her journey on the straight and narrow? Or is she back here in the city, at another hotel with a nameless man? The needle in her arm, the heroin easing her skittishness, keeping the darkness at bay, the cocaine rush making her feel invincible—is she up on the mountaintop now, her soul dancing under the stars?

CHAPTER 7

Treatment and Recovery

Addiction is a chronic disease, not an acute disease. It cannot be cured quickly like an episode of low blood sugar or a broken leg. While some people who are addicted bristle at the idea that their addiction is a disease, what can't be disputed is that the drive to use drugs is complicated, and it is difficult, if not impossible, for many to avoid. Reprogramming behaviors and repairing brains is not simple or quick, but brains and people can recover with help.

The problem for many is in getting the help. In the United States, only 22 percent of those with substance use disorder receive medication treatment. Our society too often treats addiction like a crime and punishes those addicted rather than helping them with treatment. When someone with a history of substance use relapses, many consider the relapse a moral failing. People in treatment are often kicked out of their treatment programs if they are found to have used drugs. Patients on methadone maintenance, an FDA-approved treatment for opioid use disorder, are often bounced out of the program if they are found to test positive for other drugs and are denied

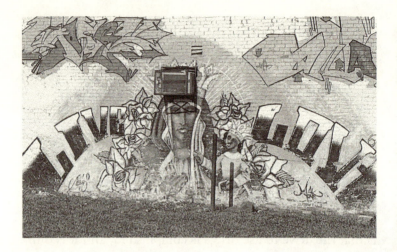

access to a drug that has been proven to help people beat addiction. Imagine a cancer patient who beat cancer five years ago being denied further chemotherapy because their cancer has been found to return. People on methadone who become incarcerated are often not allowed to stay on methadone while in prison. Diabetics don't have their insulin taken away from them when they are in prison, but for some reason, it is okay to take medicine away from people with substance use disorder. We have to stop thinking of drug use as a moral lapse.

Drug addiction is a chronic disease. People with drug addiction should be shown the same empathy people with other chronic diseases are shown. Chronic diseases such as hypertension, asthma, and drug use are treatable. Chronic diseases that are not treated often lead to preventable deaths. Once the patient has the disease, the disease causes changes in their biology that need to be addressed not on one visit but over time. Chronic diseases require long-term monitoring because **relapse is almost always part of the recovery process.** Patients with high blood pressure, diabetes, and asthma all have relapse rates as high as or higher than drug addiction relapse rates. But patients with high blood pressure, diabetes, and asthma are not punished when they relapse. Some diabetics often eat poorly and fail to follow exercise regimes. Some asthmatics smoke, and some people with hypertension eat highly salted foods. None of them are subsequently denied their medications or kicked out of wellness programs because they did not perfectly adhere to their prescribed treatment. Hypertension, diabetes, and anti-smoking programs are not punitive. Likewise, drug treatment should not be punitive. We should be doing everything we can to help people succeed. The goal of drug use treatment should be long-term survival, not punishing anyone who is not 100 percent abstinent.

DETOXIFICATION

Detoxification is a first step for those seeking to stop using drugs. Stopping outright without assistance, often called going "cold turkey," is an excruciating and sometimes life-threatening process. People often refer to opioid withdrawal as the worst flu imaginable times 100. Many who try to quit on their own cannot tolerate the severity of the withdrawal, knowing that all they have to do to feel better is to use again. Cold turkey is a barbaric way to detox and is not recommended.

Supervised detoxification under medical care is the safe way to proceed. A detoxification program should consist of three components: evaluation, stabilization, and "fostering a patient's entry into treatment." Evaluation includes testing the substances in a person's system, evaluating the patient's medical and psychological needs, and developing an individualized treatment plan. Stabilization includes using medications to safely ease the withdrawal and educating the patient and their support system into what to expect from the treatment process. Fostering a patient's entry into treatment involves getting the patient to commit to a treatment plan and may involve a nonbinding contract of expectations.

Detoxification can occur in an acute care hospital or another specialized setting. Typical detoxification lasts for seven days. Detoxification alone is not treatment, however. While it can eliminate the drug from a patient's system and clear them out so they are no longer in physical withdrawal, **detoxification does not address the body's and brain's chemical changes due to the addiction**. Detox must go hand in hand with getting a patient committed to continual treatment services.

TREATMENT PROGRAMS

No single treatment works for everyone. Treatment should be tailored to an individual's needs. Treatment programs include residential and outpatient. Residential treatment secludes the person from the outside world and involves intensive programs, including individual and group sessions, as well as various kinds of therapy, from exercise to anger management and targeted therapy for mental health issues. Inpatient programs typically last three weeks to 12 months depending on a person's needs and resources. Inpatient treatment can be very expensive. The National Center for Drug Abuse Statistics estimates the average cost for a 30-day inpatient program is $12,500.

Outpatient treatment can enable a person to continue working and living with their family. It is not as intense as inpatient treatment, but it can work for many. If a patient fails outpatient treatment, the patient can then try residential treatment. A physician should help a patient or family decide the best first course of treatment for their needs.

The two main forms of treatment are behavioral therapy and medication-assisted treatment (MAT). They can and should go in sync.

BEHAVIORAL THERAPY

Behavioral therapy includes group and individual sessions that focus on modifying a patient's behavior patterns to help them recognize situations that might lead to their renewed drug use. It teaches them how to avoid or at least cope with these situations. Patients learn to recognize what influences their drug use and work to improve their daily function, and they receive positive reinforcement for behavior changes. Effective treatment should look not just at the drug use but also at the underlying pain that may have driven someone to find relief from suffering. No simple fix. No overnight miracle. But a journey.

MEDICATION-ASSISTED TREATMENT (MAT)

MAT includes methadone, buprenorphine, and naltrexone. Methadone and buprenorphine are opioids that suppress the desire to use stronger opioids and depress withdrawal symptoms without providing the euphoria typical of opioids like heroin and fentanyl. They are difficult to overdose on. The argument has been made that people using MAT are just replacing one opioid with another. That may be true, but instead of opioids like heroin or fentanyl that kill and completely disrupt a life, methadone and buprenorphine enable people to be with their family, to work and pay taxes, and to lead productive lives. These opioids restore an equilibrium to the brain's circuits and can help lead to healing.

Methadone is usually obtained from a clinic where people are given a daily dose to drink. If they are compliant with the program, they are eventually given doses to take home between visits. People should be on methadone for at least a year before tapering off. Many are on methadone long term.

Buprenorphine works similarly but can be prescribed by a physician for take-home use. **Suboxone** is a version of the drug that includes naloxone, which is added to prevent people from misusing buprenorphine, although buprenorphine misuse is rare.

Naltrexone is an extended-release nonopioid that blocks opioid receptors and prevents people from getting high. It can only be given once someone has completed detoxification.

Medication-assisted treatment includes one of these medications and therapy to help resolve a patient's negative behavior patterns. Patients who have completed initial drug treatment, whether behavioral or medication assisted, should be followed by health workers and undergo continued therapy and support to mitigate relapse risks. These drugs and treatments have been proven to combat addiction. Up to 90 percent of people on MAT stay sober for at least two years. When buprenorphine was introduced in Baltimore in 1995, it was credited with decreasing heroin deaths by 37 percent over the next 15 years. In addition to reducing fatal overdoses, MAT has been shown to decrease illicit opioid use, keep people in treatment, and improve people's ability to get and maintain work, as well as reduce the risk of contracting HIV and hepatitis C.

Unfortunately, neither methadone nor buprenorphine, which are considered essential medicines by the World Health Organization, are available in the numbers needed to treat the millions of Americans who suffer with opioid use disorder (OUD). Only 36.5 percent of those with OUD received any treatment in 2021, and only 22.3 percent received medications. Imagine if insulin was available to only one out of five people with diabetes or hypertension drugs to only one out of five people with high blood pressure. It would be a national shame. I can think of no comparable conditions where medications proven to be so effective in saving lives are so sparsely available. Unfortunately, government red tape and stigma are to blame for the lack of easy availability for these important medications.

BUPRENORPHINE BARRIERS

Until recently, any physician with a DEA license could prescribe prescription opioids to patients, but only those with a special "X waiver" could prescribe buprenorphine. For instance, say you were in pain. Your family physician could write you a prescription for oxycodone to ease the pain, and as your tolerance grew, he could increase your dosage and extend your prescription. But if you were to become addicted, as so many have, he could not write you a prescription for a drug proven to effectively treat your disorder. He would have to send you to a specialist who had an X waiver, and for a time, even doctors with X waivers could only treat a finite number of patients with buprenorphine. A survey showed that other physician barriers to prescribing buprenorphine included lack of institutional support, concern about their own lack of training to manage opioid use disorder, and lack of treatment services. The DEA finally did away with both the X waiver and the limited number of patients a physician could treat with buprenorphine. Additionally, physicians can now prescribe buprenorphine via telemedicine, an initiative that began during COVID and proved effective without any of the worries that had prohibited it before the pandemic.

METHADONE BARRIERS

A significant barrier to methadone treatment is how inconvenient it is to obtain. Patients can't go to their pharmacy to pick it up. They must travel (sometimes a great distance) five to six times a week to a licensed facility and often wait in a long line that may extend outside the building until they can get to the window and be handed their dose, which they have to drink in front of a provider. (In Hartford, there is a methadone clinic on Main Street, and anyone driving to work can see the faces of those standing in line outside the building.)

Childcare and unreliable transportation can prove difficult obstacles to getting and maintaining this evidence-based treatment. If people don't arrive on time, the door is locked, with no admittance to stragglers. I have responded to several overdoses for patients who missed the morning methadone cutoff and instead bought opioids on the street to ease their cravings. I once responded to a person in a car accident who refused ambulance transport despite an obvious broken wrist so he could get to the methadone clinic before it closed. Studies have shown that methadone treatment is also more concentrated in poor areas with higher minority populations, while buprenorphine is more likely to be prescribed to better-off white patients. Methadone is highly stigmatized. And the costs can be unaffordable to the poor. Unaffordability can only be corrected by changing the laws to permanently have Medicare and Medicaid cover all OUD medications and treatment, to enable methadone to be provided in office settings, and to allow it to be picked up at pharmacies.

NALTREXONE

Naltrexone, unlike methadone or buprenorphine, is not an opioid and therefore has no potential for abuse. It works by blocking the opioid receptors and thus preventing people who use opioids from getting high. There is some controversy over whether naltrexone reduces cravings in opioid-abstinent people. It is only intended for people who are no longer dependent on opioids. If given to someone who is dependent, it will cause withdrawal. It should be used with behavioral therapy. It can be given as a pill or an extended-release injection once a month, though the injection is recommended due to lower compliance with the pill regime.

WHAT TO LOOK FOR IN TREATMENT OPTIONS

There are many sad stories of people being swindled by drug treatment centers that lack sufficient medical oversight and trained staff. People who break small rules can be summarily kicked to the street. The nonprofit organization Shatterproof, founded by Gary Mendell, a father who lost his son to addiction, recently proposed a set of principles to guide people to care that is aligned with clinical standards of care. According to Shatterproof, quality addiction treatment should include "fast access to treatment, personalized evaluation and treatment plan, access to medications for opioid or alcohol use disorder, effective behavioral therapies for addiction, long-term treatment and follow-up, coordinated care for mental and physical health, additional services to support recovery, and routine screenings in every medical setting."

Shatterproof is going state by state and creating a directory of addiction treatment sites to help people find the best treatment for their unique needs. They recently launched their resource in Connecticut, making it the fifteenth state in which they have accomplished this. Mendell tells a moving story of love and sadness at his inability to help his son Brian, who went to rehab eight times and who he said died not of overdose but of suicide caused by his shame over his addiction and failure to overcome it. The group Mendell founded is dedicated to improving treatment options by ending the stigma that kills every bit as much as the drugs.

According to the CDC, OUD cost the country $1.02 trillion in 2017, counting law enforcement, health care costs, substance use treatment, loss of life, and loss of productivity. Of this, $14.8 billion was spent on law enforcement, while only $3.5 billion was spent on treatment. We need to reorient our priorities.

Pink Froth

Our unconscious patient's chest heaves again, and he coughs up another gob of high-flying trapeze pink froth that splats on the ambulance bench seat where seconds before my partner's knee had been. As he secures the IV, I check the patient's pupils. Midsize, unreactive. No one home.

Ten minutes before, bystanders who found the man slumped forward in the car gave him Narcan and pulled him out onto the pavement. They said he wasn't breathing, he had pinpoint pupils, and there were syringes on the seat. He is a big man and was difficult to lift up onto the stretcher, dead weight. We don't need to ventilate him anymore with the bag-valve mask as he is breathing 14 times a minute, and he is no longer blue and dusky. His oxygen saturation is 92 percent, so I put him on an oxygen mask, periodically removing it to suction the froth.

No one knew how long he was parked there. He no doubt bought his fentanyl on Park Street, then headed west, pulling into this shopping plaza and parking in the first available spot—a spot where I have responded to several overdoses in the past. When he went out, his glottis, the opening between his vocal chords likely closed, and his body, trying to breath against his now-occluded airway, created extra pressure that damaged the alveoli in his lungs, causing this pink froth that is filling the bottom of our suction canister.

His driver's license says he is from a Connecticut town down by the shore, but when we put his name in our laptop, an address of a transient motel on the Berlin Turnpike comes up, the kind of motel where we routinely call the time on residents found dead by the motel staff. In his wallet are school photos of a young boy; each of the three photos are of the same kid, one year older than the last, maybe third, fourth, and fifth grade, guessing. No pictures of a mom. Business cards for a methadone clinic and a probation officer.

I wonder who will get calls from the hospital telling them what is going on. Will any family member or friend sit in the ICU waiting room for updates as he lies in a bed intubated and sedated with a likely anoxic brain injury? And how many others like him today are in the same situation? Alveoli burst under the stress of trying to breath against a closed airway. Naloxone rushing to the brain. Bubbling pink froth flying through the air to be wiped away or end up in soon-to-be-discarded suction canisters after they have been wheeled into another ED. Meanwhile, broken families try to go about their lives. Telephones no longer carry the voices of those they loved.

CHAPTER 8

Harm Reduction

Keeping People Alive

I had been a paramedic for 20 years before I even heard the term *harm reduction*. As a paramedic, my job was to respond to an emergency, treat that emergency, and take the patient to the hospital. If it was an overdose, I might throw in my two cents to the patient about the need to stop doing drugs before they ended up dead or in jail, but the advice wasn't part of the job. Some progressive EMS systems were starting to change the way they looked at some emergencies. If you were in a house that had fall hazards such as loose rugs, you might point them out. If a patient was a diabetic, you might talk with them about diet, exercise, and the need to regularly take their medications. Kids riding bicycles were told to wear helmets. People riding in cars were encouraged to wear seat belts. Some EMS personnel learned how to properly install child safety seats and to share that information with families they encountered on the job. Commonsense stuff. All these things prevented harm. I never imagined that I would one day tell

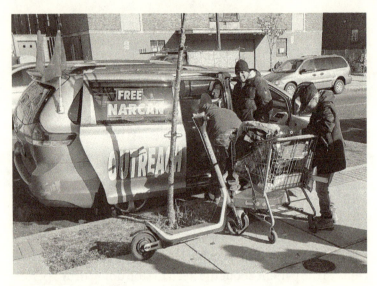

Harm reduction outreach

patients whom I had resuscitated from overdose how to use drugs safely if they chose to use again.

When we in EMS first heard that laypeople were going to start using naloxone, many of us shook our heads. Even when it was proposed that first responders could carry naloxone, there was resistance from paramedics. First responders didn't have the education and advanced assessment skills that paramedics did to judge what was an opioid overdose and what wasn't. And what if the naloxone puts the patient into pulmonary edema, a rare side effect? Paramedics carried medications to combat pulmonary edema; basic first responders didn't. Fortunately, good judgment prevailed, and not only did laypeople start administering naloxone, but soon so did police, firefighters, and basic-level emergency medical technicians. The truth was that opioid overdoses were easy to diagnose, and the harm from administering naloxone was exceedingly small and far outweighed by the benefits. Today, more than half the time I respond to an opioid overdose, someone—a bystander, a police officer, or a firefighter—has already given naloxone. Sometimes I have responded to "the unconscious person" only to find no one on scene, just an empty vial of naloxone. The unconscious person revived and was well enough to flee the approaching sirens.

I once attended an overdose prevention conference where a man named Mark Jenkins talked about harm reduction. He struck me as someone speaking the truth. He said the job of harm reduction was to save lives because dead people aren't able to make good decisions. I began to see Mark and the people he worked with out on the streets of Hartford. Sometimes they would be at overdose scenes before me or arrive shortly after. If a layperson had given naloxone and was still there, I would ask them where they got the naloxone, and they would often answer they'd gotten it from Mark or from his organization, the Greater Hartford Harm Reduction Coalition.

Mark's group eventually opened The Drop on Albany Avenue in an area where drug use and overdoses were common. People go to this drop-in center for syringe exchange, to get naloxone, or to find help with services if they are ready for that. The center also has a shower people can use. They even serve sandwiches. Some people just like sitting in there and talking. Eventually Mark hired a nurse to help people with their wounds, give vaccines, and provide medical testing. The Drop is a safe place for people who often fall through the gaps. Mark also installed a bathroom with a door that swings out instead of in so that it can be accessed from the outside. People can do whatever they want in the bathroom, but they have to give their name to the staff member at the desk across from the door, who sets a timer. After three minutes, the person knocks on the door and asks if everything is okay. If someone overdoses in the bathroom, the staff revives them with naloxone. I have responded there several times for overdoses, and when I'd arrive, the person would already be alert and breathing. Sometimes I'd take them to the hospital; other times the staff would sit with them until they were well enough to leave. No one has died in Mark's bathroom, unlike the people we have found dead in the locked bathrooms of the fast-food restaurants on the avenue or in the Porta Potties in the nearby park.

Currently the federal crack house statute prevents anyone from running buildings for the purposes of people consuming illegal drugs. The crack house statute was designed to stop landlords who knowingly ran crack houses and shooting galleries where many people overdosed and died. It was not intended to, but in effect prevented people from legally establishing overdose prevention sites for legitimate public health reasons. That said, the justice department under President Joe Biden, who actually wrote the crack house statute as a much younger man, did not enforce this provision against public health sites. They also did not enforce the federal laws against marijuana possession, which is legal under many state laws. Whether or not the justice department in the new Trump administration will change course is unknown as of the writing of this book

In June 2022, I spoke on a panel with Sam Rivera, the man who started and runs New York City's two supervised injection sites. In just a few months of operation, the New York facilities served over a thousand people. The most interesting part of his talk was his description of the camaraderie that has developed among the people who use drugs there. Instead of doing an extra bag, people are talking with each other about the NBA finals. Women who avoided mirrors when they started coming there are now wearing makeup. The place is a community where people feel safe, respected for who they are, and yes, loved. People no longer see themselves as junkies, the objects of scorn and stigma, but as Dougs, Rogers, Sylvias, Marias, and Pattis. People are called by their given names, not by generic slurs. While they are there, they can shower. The staff will do their laundry and provide clean underwear for some. The people feel respected, human. These supervised injection sites are not just a place where people can use drugs safely, but as the harm reduction activist Guy Felicella has said, they're "also a place to *stop* using drugs." People are there to help get people who use drugs into detox and recovery when they are ready.

Mark and Sam Rivera and their brethren in harm reduction don't question, "Am I my brother's keeper?" They live their lives and do their chosen work with love for their fellow travelers on this earth. Whether they believe in an afterlife or in nothingness, they are holy people deserving of our greatest reverence in a world that is no stranger to greed and hate.

Mark introduced me to a friend of his, Van Asher, a former EMT and current harm reductionist, who creates educational videos. In one called "Harm Reduction and Abstinence Based Treatment, 'Bridging the Gap,'" Asher describes harm reduction as a life raft that rescues people in the sea. Harm reduction helps some people make it to shore (treatment), and for others who choose to live in the sea, it keeps them from drowning. Harm reduction bridges the gap between active use and treatment.

Typical harm reduction services include counseling, naloxone distribution, syringe exchange and safe-use supplies (cookers, saline bullets, alcohol wipes, cotton to filter out impurities, clean tourniquets), fentanyl test strips and drug-checking services, safe-sex supplies, safe-smoking supplies (safe mouthpieces with filters to prevent burns), antibiotic ointments, wound treatment, vitamin C to help prevent infections and promote healing, food, clothes, and even from organizations like Mark's, tents and sleeping bags for the homeless if Mark's group is unable to find them shelter.

At the hospital I bring in an overdose patient whom we have resuscitated with naloxone. While the nurse has him change into a hospital gown, I see a security guard going through his backpack. He sees a package of syringes and takes them out and throws them into the trash.

"What are you doing?" I say. "Those are his."

"It's against our policy," he replies.

"You can't throw his stuff away."

"The hell I can't."

"Hold on a minute," I tell him. I find a young ED doctor and explain what is going on. "When this guy gets out of the hospital and he's going to need to use again, and he's not going to have his clean syringes, he's going to pick one off the ground or share one with someone and he's going to get AIDS, hep C, or endocarditis. They give out clean syringes to prevent this from happening." The doctor then intervenes with the security guard, and the syringes along with the backpack are safely stored. I tell Mark about this encounter, and he later meets with hospital representatives and starts providing them with safe-use kits that they can give to people who are being discharged. I like Mark because he is a no-bullshit, make-ithappen guy. He is on the street and brings those voices with him when he meets with committees and government employees who are often on longer time schedules. There is not a lot of patience for tabling discussion till next month's meeting when people are dying every day. Mark understands and is able to convey that urgency.

Harm reduction is concerned first and foremost with saving lives. Moral judgments are cast aside. The message is that people matter. Harm reduction enables people to use safely until they are ready to quit. Instead of promoting drug use, harm reduction ultimately results in less drug use and more people getting into treatment. It means less death.

Harm reduction is also cost efficient. Studies have shown that for every dollar spent on syringe exchange, six dollars is saved in treating HIV costs. The savings is even higher if you factor in the costs of treating hepatitis C infections. Syringe exchange has also been proven to increase entry into treatment, further saving millions in health and economic costs.

A study published in *The Lancet* in 2016 compared the overdose rate of a Vancouver neighborhood in the two years before the opening of the safe-injection site, Insite, with the rate in the two years after Insite opened and found that it had decreased by 35 percent. Other studies showed that the supervised injection site had led to a greater chance of users getting off drugs and to increased use of treatment services.

A cost-benefit analysis of how much a similar safe-injection site would benefit Baltimore, Maryland, which has one of the worst overdose death rates in the country, was published in the *Harm Reduction Journal* in 2017. The study looked at six different benefits: preventing the spread of HIV, hepatitis C, skin and soft-tissue infections, and overdose deaths; decreasing costs associated with nonfatal overdoses; and enabling people to get into MAT. The study found that for an investment of $1.8 million, a safe-injection site would save $7.8 million in costs, prevent deaths, reduce infections, limit days spent in a hospital for skin infections, reduce ambulance runs, decrease ED use and hospital admission, and get more people into treatment.

Harm reduction won't cure homelessness, hunger, poverty, racism, unequal educational opportunity, or any of the other social ills that can lead to despair and substance use, but it clearly helps keep people alive, particularly those who easily fall through the gaps. That's no small achievement.

A Ravine in Winter

There is a picture in the Hartford Courant *of Mark Jenkins talking with police officers, looking as forlorn as I have ever seen him. They stand next to yellow tape sectioning off an area of woods just off Park Terrace, where down a small ravine a man has been found dead. The paper describes the crime scene as a homeless encampment, but it is little more than a small clearing with a dirty mattress, a blanket over some branches acting as a tarpaulin, and a hollowed-out log. Mark is the leader of the Greater Hartford Harm Reduction Coalition. A former user who went to rehab himself 17 times. With the help of friends, he found his way and now has dedicated his life to harm reduction.*

A couple of months back, I got dispatched to this same place for an overdose. Mark and two members of his organization, José and Bryan, were already there. They had been on their way to work on the construction of their new walk-in center when they were flagged down. They found a man cold and not breathing on the broken winter branches and mat of old heroin bags. They gave him naloxone, and by the time I arrived, the man was breathing again. He was just starting to rouse and was combative in his haze. They helped us carry him up to our stretcher. He was lucky someone had seen him and that Mark and his crew were driving by. In the hospital the man's core temperature was 90 degrees.

Some days when I am working, I stop by the site. A few weeks ago, after we'd pulled to the side of the road, I looked down the small ravine and saw a solitary man there. From my vantage, I saw he had his arm outstretched and was injecting himself. In the summertime, the clearing is completely hidden by greenery, but in winter, it is all gray and naked trees. The man nevertheless blended in in jeans and a black shirt, as if in this same season, he had stripped himself of much of what he once was.

I don't know if the dead man is the same man I took to the hospital or the man I saw injecting himself in the cold grayness or another similar lost soul. I do know that he is not the first to die in those woods.

In Mark's face, you can see the burden of this war he is fighting against stigma, against convention and bureaucracy, against death, against time.

CHAPTER 9

The Harms of Stigma

Naloxone will not save you if you use alone. I have found naloxone on many of the overdose death scenes I have been on. Often it is within reach of the body. Ninety-one percent of people who die from opioid overdoses die using alone. Why do they use alone? Stigma. Stigma causes people to hide their addiction. The stigma of being an "addict" implies that person is to blame for their actions. The words we use to describe someone affect not only how we view that person but also how that person comes to view themselves. Stigma prevents people from seeking help.

When I started working as a paramedic, others told me about the junkies and addicts I would encounter. These were people who, rather than living the norms of society, were members of an estranged group that was a drag on the rest of us. They were "dirty," while those who didn't use were "clean." Health care and other public money spent on them, including our time, was considered a waste because it was unnecessary and due only to their bad character. Our taxes were higher because of their weakness.

THE HARMS OF STIGMA

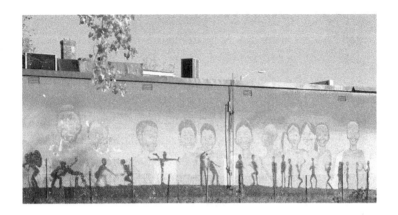

My coworkers, like many people in emergency health care, including doctors, were never well trained, if trained at all, in addiction, mental health, or the dangers of stigma. We passed on a culture biased against drug users that had been passed on to us. For a while, I carried the torch.

My friend Kelley is a heroin and cocaine user. I have known her for around a decade now, and she has helped me understand a lot about the epidemic. When I met her, early in her addiction, I was surprised to learn that she used drugs at all. She was a bright, clear-complexioned twenty-something with purple hair and half her head shaved, sort of a punk-girl-next-door type. She suffered from anxiety and came from an unstable household. Her mother, who was addicted to pills, would give Kelley Percocets for her menstrual cramps and migraines. Her path led to heroin and homelessness.

Later, when she had bad abscesses on her arms and legs, I urged her, as I often did, to go to the hospital with me and get checked out, get treatment for her wounds, and maybe even get into rehab again or get on Suboxone or methadone. They could help her there, I said. But she'd just shake her head. "They treated me like shit the time I overdosed. They don't like me there. I will never go back to the hospital." I heard similar stories from others I knew. What upset me the most was when one user told me how she was treated by one of my fellow medics, who said to her, "I'm tired of scraping your ass off the pavement." Both 911 scenes and the ED were not welcoming places for them. They felt judged there, and so barring being unresponsive, they did everything they could to avoid going there. I was thrilled when the local harm reduction group opened a drop-in center and staffed it with a nurse whom I could send them to see. She could treat them and do her best to get them the care they needed.

The word *stigma* means "stain." When we stigmatize someone, we put a stain on them. It suggests not just moral judgment against a person, but it also inspires fear in others, works to isolate people, and criminalizes their behavior. The user becomes a stereotype and not a person. A "dope fiend" is not someone considered capable of positive human interaction.

The World Health Organization studied stigma in 14 countries to determine what conditions (homelessness, AIDS, obesity, mental disorders, alcoholism, criminal record for burglary, etc.) were most likely to be stigmatized. Drug use was number one.

On TV and on the news, the images that accompany stories on the drug crisis often show people living in squalor, rooting through garbage cans, and trying to inject their necks or feet. Their drug use in public is portrayed as a crime, not the result of a disease and social situation. Headlines blame addicts for unsafe streets rather than focusing on homelessness and mental health. People who use drugs are often seen as inhuman. A recent article about drug use in San Francisco drew the headline "Zombie Apocalypse." Who wants to read about human tragedy and unaddressed social needs when zombie terror gets all the clicks?

On YouTube there are plentiful stereotype-reinforcing videos, such as one that has received over a million views titled "Skin Rotting 'Zombie Drug' Causes Havoc Across the US," which portrays drug users like characters in horror stories, complete with terrifying ominous soundtracks. Local news stations covering the crisis typically show footage of people using drugs near dumpsters. The term *junkie* came from "junk men," people who went through trash. The association is that junkies are human trash.

One day I was dispatched to an overdose. I was in the paramedic rapid response car, and a BLS crew was in the ambulance. We were driving around looking for the victim. I didn't see anyone on two passes, but then I heard the BLS unit radio that they'd found the patient. I swung around to where they were now parked at the curb with their lights still flashing. An EMT was already wheeling the stretcher down a short alley, where his partner knelt by the dumpster. As I approached, I saw he had the bag-valve-mask out and was providing ventilations to a man who was dusky with agonal respirations.

"Thought I'd check behind the dumpster," the EMT said to me.

"You found him." I marveled at his simple logic.

In EMS when we meet people with OUD, we often find them at rock bottom. I have responded to many overdoses like this one of people who were down alleys and behind dumpsters. From TV news coverage, many would assume that all drug users seek out trash cans to hide behind while they stick "dirty" needles in their scab- and abscessed-filled wasted arms. The young EMT did, and it helped us find this lost soul.

Rock bottom means there is no lower that someone can go. It is a common belief that someone needs to hit rock bottom before they are ready for help. I think of my early remarks to the users I revived before I thought to ask them their stories, when I just saw them as people who needed to get a grip. "Get your life together, just say no, or you are going to end up dead or in jail. Look at yourself." I held up to them not a picture of who they could be again but who society saw them as—junkies, human trash. It is hard enough to make something of yourself in this world, much less when your current position is at rock bottom with the world looking down on you.

Stereotypes produce negative judgments, and negative judgments lead to discrimination. Would you give a job or rent an apartment to a "drug abuser"? Would you give a sandwich and some change to a "zombie"? If you were a legislator, would you allocate money to an "abuser" that instead could go to someone who is not an "abuser"?

Language affects how society feels about people who use drugs; it also affects how people who use drugs feel about themselves. Steven Biko, the great South African human rights leader, said, "The most potent weapon in the hands of the oppressor is the mind of the oppressed." If you can destroy a man's self-worth, you can cripple his ability to stand up.

Say you have just overdosed. A large first responder with a military-style crew cut and bull-sized chest stands over you and barks, "Tell me what drugs you used. How many bags? What's wrong with you? You're going to kill yourself. Think of your family. Get some self-respect. I'm being honest with you, bro, keeping it real. You're a mess. Look in the mirror. You're at rock bottom."

Do you want to be in this person's care? Do you want to go to the hospital and be lectured by people who also think you are a scumbag? You are an abuser. You are a junkie. The triage nurse who is scolding you has a coffee mug that says, "The

Tears of My Drug-Seekers." How does that make you feel? What are you going to do? Everyone looks down on you. You just want to crawl back into your own hole. You want to forget. Even if someone was there to help you, you would likely just mess it up again. With no one else to turn to, you turn back to the needle. Your only friend. The damage is done.

Not only do we need to help people at rock bottom; we need to start helping them before they get there.

Science has shown that social pain is felt in the same area of the brain as physical pain and thus responds to pain medicine in the same way physical pain responds. In an opinion piece in the *New England Journal of Medicine*, Dr. Nora Volkow cites a study in which lab rats chose interacting with other lab rats over self-administering drugs, but when they were punished with electrical shocks for their social interactions, they reverted to drug use. She concludes that stigma "spurs further drug taking."

People who use drugs hide their use for fear of being stigmatized. They are worried they will lose the respect of others as well as cost themselves economically. It is hard to seek treatment for a problem that you don't want the world to see. Even when people do need to get medical treatment for either the disease or its after effects, they may not be treated as other people seeking medical attention are due to the negative views many health care providers have about people who use drugs.

Anti-stigma advocates are working hard to get the media to pay attention to the language they use. The Associated Press's stylebook now attempts to steer media people in the right direction, urging them to avoid stigmatizing or punitive words that can deter people from seeking treatment. Instead of *abuse* or *problems*, reporters are encouraged to use the words *use* or *misuse*. They are warned to avoid the words *addict*, *abuser*, *junkie*, and *crackhead*. These words stereotype and dehumanize rather than recognize the humanity of the person with the medical condition.

Recently the *Hartford Courant* ran a story about xylazine, the animal tranquilizer that is being used as an adulterant to fentanyl and can cause skin lesions and necrotic wounds. The headline of the story on their website read, "'Modern Day Leprosy': Xylazine Hits Connecticut with Devastating Impact." For people who only read news headlines this stigmatizing language is damaging. I emailed the reporter, who likely was not the one responsible for the headline, and wrote, "Calling xylazine wounds leprosy (I know it's a catchy quote) can be very stigmatizing and may keep some people from providing aid to overdose victims for fear of catching 'modern day leprosy.' Xylazine wounds are not contagious." The paper's website changed the headline to read, "Zombie Drug Hits Connecticut with Devastating Impact."

In a December 2023 article in the *Atlantic*, Keith Humphreys and Jonathan Caulkins argue that the United States must walk the line between destigmatizing drug addiction, which they see as a noble endeavor, and destigmatizing drug use, which they see as dangerous. They argue that harm reduction campaigns that encourage people to "do it with friends" rather than use alone "promote a positive image of a drug that is killing 200 Americans a day." They argue that harm reduction is geared toward people who are already using and that we must consider people who have not yet started if we want to truly end the epidemic. They approve of campaigns like "One Pill Can Kill" and cite how stigma has helped curtail smoking by deglamorizing it. I disagree that harm reduction glamorizes drug use. Its foremost concern is saving human lives. One of the National Harm Reduction Coalition's eight Principles of Harm Reduction is "Does not attempt to minimize or ignore the real and tragic harm and danger that can be associated with illicit drug use."

Ending stigma could change the course of this epidemic. People who use drugs are human beings knocked off course by a larger epidemic not of their making. None of them set out to become addicted to drugs, to become homeless, or to lose their families or their lives. An addictive gene, an accident, a doctor's prescription, an innocent experimentation, a history of sexual abuse, or mental health problems, diagnosed or undiagnosed—so many factors are behind their use. We must stop driving people into the shadows or locking them up because we don't like their disease. Drug treatment, housing, health care, job support, human empathy, and love will go further than hurtful words and prison bars. As humans, we all belong to each other.

We need to truthfully educate people about drug use. Scare tactics are not as effective as plain truth. Cut the zombie nonsense, and tell it like it is. Fentanyl kills. People who use illicit opioids must know that they cannot effectively judge the dose. People who buy illicit pills must know that those pills may not be what they say they are; they may contain a lethal dose of fentanyl. People who use illicit drugs should never use alone. Fentanyl plus using alone is deadly. That is truth.

A Confrontation

We get called for a woman in withdrawal seeking detox. She is at a bus stop with all her belongings stuffed into two large garbage bags. We get her on a stretcher and carry her bags with us to the ambulance. She is aching and has abdominal pain and nausea. It has been 12 hours since she last used. And however bad she is feeling now, she knows it's only going to get worse. "Will they treat me okay there?" she asks me.

"I hope so," I say.

"A couple of the nurses don't like me."

"Maybe they won't be working, and at any rate, even if they are not as nice as they could be, you'll have a place to rest for a little while and get something to eat."

"I'm not hungry," she says. She looks miserable.

"Well, you can at least rest."

We talk on the way there. I learn that she broke her back in a car accident 20 years ago when she was 17. Once her doctor cut her off from Percocet, she bought pills on the street. It took her only nine months to turn to heroin, which has been her captor ever since. She has been on the streets for most of the last 15 years. She can't remember the number of times she's been in rehab.

When we get to the ED, I go to the triage desk and give my report. The nurse looks over at the woman on our stretcher. "Ah, our friend Carol," she says. "Has she been difficult for you?"

"No, perfectly fine."

The nurse nods. "She was here last week for abdominal pain, looking for pain meds. When I said she had to sit in the waiting room and wait her turn, she went spider monkey on me. Security had to throw her out."

"She's in no shape to fight anyone right now," I say, understanding that sometimes users who are in withdrawal and seeking drugs can let their irritability turn into bad behavior. It is not uncommon to hear users and nurses cuss each other out. The nurses are struggling to place patients without enough beds available, and the users, in the throes of withdrawal, want to stop feeling sick. They want someone to acknowledge the hell going on inside their body. When they get what they perceive as a callous or uncaring response, they can react badly.

I walk with the nurse over to our stretcher. "Remember me?" the nurse says to Carol. Two muscled security guards stand behind the nurse with their arms crossed. There is something about the nurse's tone and stance that reminds me of a prison warden.

"Oh, fuck," Carol says. "She's the one I was talking about."

"Hello, Carol," the nurse says. "Are you going to behave, or are we going to have to restrain you?"

"I'm sick," the woman says, quietly.

"You know we are awfully busy here today."

"I'm sick," she says again, but more tensely.

I start shaking my head. I have seen this scene play out many times before, and it seems so unnecessary.

"Are you going to sit quietly until it's your turn?"

"Fuck you," Carol says.

The scene quickly deteriorates and ends with Carol tied, screaming, to a bed in four-point restraints.

CHAPTER 10

Ending the War on People/ Hope for the Future

If telling people "just say no or you are going to end up dead or in jail" worked, then there would be no opioid epidemic today. If putting people—many addicted to drugs themselves—in jail for life for dealing $3 bags of fentanyl worked, there would be no fentanyl available to buy on the street. Unfortunately, these strategies fail. Demanding abstinence and locking up people for low-level drug offenses has done nothing more than fill up our cemeteries and penitentiaries.

Supreme Court Justice William O. Douglas in a landmark ruling in Robinson v. California, wrote, "It is cruel and unusual punishment in the sense of the eighth amendment to treat as a criminal a person who is a drug addict." You cannot treat a disease as a crime and expect to eradicate it.

In a June 2023 story in the *New York Times*, reporter Eli Saslow tells the story of two friends who while waiting to get into detox purchase $30 worth of fentanyl to ward off the sickness of drug withdrawal. Both use the drug. They both

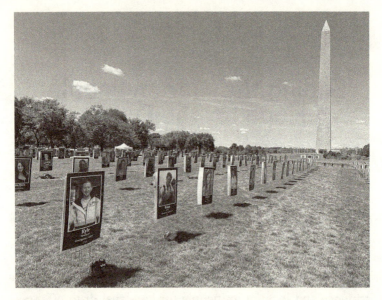

Today I Matter poster memorial at National Mall honoring 640 lost family members

nod off. When one comes around, he notices the other is not responsive. He drives frantically to a nearby gas station, asks them to call 911, and does CPR on his friend until the paramedics arrive. The conscious man, who has a 25-year history of addiction that began with a prescription following a car accident and PTSD stemming from being raped as a 9-year-old, is charged with first-degree murder for obtaining the fentanyl. Nothing happens to the dealer he bought the fentanyl from.

Instead of going to rehab while awaiting trial, he goes to jail, where drugs are so widely available that he overdoses and needs to be revived with naloxone himself. No charges are filed against the warden for running a drug-ridden jail. The man, who could have avoided all this trouble by abandoning his friend instead of trying to save his life, takes a plea deal to first-degree manslaughter to avoid a life sentence.

Pounding the podium and declaring yourself tough on drugs may make for rally cheers and election-day votes, but it is not showing results on the streets. I understand the urge and frustration. Why can't you just stop using drugs? Why?! Science tells us why. Addiction is caused by a combination of genetics and environmental factors. People with substance use disorder have a chemical imbalance in their brain that causes them to act against their self-interest. As I've mentioned, you can put people with substance use disorder in an MRI machine and see the damage in their brains in the same way you can use medical imaging to see damaged hearts and broken bones. Putting them in prison doesn't cure them of their disease.

Not one of my patients woke up and decided they wanted to throw their lives away to live homeless and hungry in American alleys and backstreets, scurrying into the shadows to avoid the law and the shame of stigma set upon them. The heads of the pharmaceutical companies who lied to the American public about the dangers of opioids, setting this whole terrible epidemic into motion, still have their mansions and yachts while many of their poor victims lie under the dirt or sit behind bars, jailed only for petty crimes and public nuisance. Sadly, there are two Americas in this epidemic: one of power and money, the other downtrodden and scapegoated. Blame the drug users, the pharmaceutical companies said to deflect from their own greed for profits.

In 2017, the opioid epidemic cost the country $1.02 trillion in health care and law enforcement spending, plus loss of life and productivity. The United States spent only $3.5 billion on treatment. Albert Einstein has been attributed to defining insanity as doing the same thing you have always done and expecting different results. That quote sums up the 50-year drug war.

Hear this now. The War on Drugs has failed. After 50 years and trillions spent, drugs are cheaper, more lethal, and more readily available than they have ever been. And before anyone claims the war represents the moral high ground, we need to look at how the war started and understand that the motives were based on politics and not reasoned policy.

John Ehrlichman, President Richard Nixon's chief of staff, confessed to a journalist the true motivation behind the War on Drugs, which began in 1971 when Nixon declared drug use "public enemy number one."

> You want to know what this was really all about? The Nixon campaign in 1968, and the Nixon White House

after that, had two enemies: the antiwar left and black people. You understand what I'm saying? We knew we couldn't make it illegal to be either against the war or black, but by getting the public to associate the hippies with marijuana and blacks with heroin. And then criminalizing both heavily, we could disrupt those communities. We could arrest their leaders, raid their homes, break up their meetings, and vilify them night after night on the evening news. Did we know we were lying about the drugs? Of course we did.

Under Ronald Reagan's presidency from 1981 to 1989, drug laws became even more punitive. Instead of going after the supply and focusing their efforts on stopping international drug cartels and organized crime, the Reagan administration went after demand. With agreement from Congress, Republicans, and Democrats, they imposed stricter sentencing on people caught using drugs, including mandatory minimum sentences, further criminalizing addiction. The new standards disproportionately affected minorities and destroyed the futures of countless individuals. Nowhere was this more apparent than with their differentiation between crack cocaine favored in the Black community and powdered cocaine celebrated on Wall Street. The two drugs were chemically essentially the same, but the punishment for crack was 100 times more severe. Possession of 5 g of crack meant a mandatory five-year sentence, while you would have to possess 500 g of powdered cocaine to get the same sentence. Although African Americans represented only 15 percent of the country's drug users in 2006, they represented 74 percent of those sentenced to prison for a drug offense. According to the National Institute on Drug Abuse, 85 percent of the prison population either has a substance use problem or were jailed for crimes involving drugs or drug use. A conviction on someone's record can make them ineligible for public housing and student aid and deny them job opportunities, making it very difficult to integrate back into society.

A chilling footnote to the incarcerations of drug users is that very few receive treatment for their addiction while in prison. Inmates get detoxed, but their underlying triggers are not addressed. Worse yet, most prisoners who were on methadone or buprenorphine before they were incarcerated stop receiving the lifesaving medication when the jail door locks them in. When they get out of prison and return to their old environment, many relapse. With decreased tolerance, they have the highest risk of fatal overdose. A study in the *New England Journal of Medicine* found that prisoners in Washington state were 12 times more likely to die in their first two weeks after release than were members of the general population (matched for age, sex, and race). Tellingly, the ex-cons were 129 times more likely to die of an overdose.

Do these drug laws have any effect on the availability and use of drugs? No. A recent research study in the *International*

Journal of Drug Policy suggests that new laws charging drug dealers with homicide will have little effect and might even have the unintended consequence of deterring people from calling 911 to report an overdose. Many dealers support their own habit by selling to others in their circle. Research found that 70 percent of state prisoners and 59 percent of federal prisoners arrested for drug trafficking were drug dependent in the month before they committed their crimes. Knowing that selling to someone who overdoses could lead to imprisonment, one friend might leave an acquaintance overdosed and alone rather than risk summoning help that could lead to a 20-year prison term.

Newspapers commonly run pictures of drug busts, showing tables with drugs piled high alongside several handguns and stacks of cash. In press releases the law enforcement spokespeople boast of getting the drugs off the street and making the community safer. Yet a recent study in the *American Journal of Public Health* showed how disruption in the drug supply often leads to even more drug overdoses. The researchers found that fatal overdoses increased in the three weeks after large drug seizures, including doubling within seven days. Unable to access their usual supply, users were forced to seek out new suppliers, whose product may have been of higher potency. Additionally, users who were unable to use for a period of time had lower tolerance when they found a new source and were therefore more prone to overdosing.

A 2020 Brookings Institution paper, "Enforcement Strategies for Fentanyl and Other Synthetic Opioids," admits that the ease with which fentanyl can be trafficked due its high lethality for small volume makes traditional law enforcement interdiction approaches destined to fail. It suggests that law enforcement's first goal should be to reduce the toxicity of the supply. In areas that are entrenched with fentanyl, they suggest targeting dealers who are careless about the inconsistency of their supply or who deal in the most potent opioids, such as carfentanil, over dealers who traffic in a supply with a more consistent dose. Dealers selling counterfeit pills disguised as common prescription drugs would also have bigger targets on their backs, as would those who allowed fentanyl to contaminate their cocaine supplies. In areas that are not yet penetrated with fentanyl (fewer and fewer markets), they suggest targeting dealers who traffic in fentanyl above those who sell heroin. This could also be done on an international level, severely punishing drug organizations that traffic in fentanyl while being more permissive with those that sell heroin. There is early evidence that this approach may be having some effect based on reports that the Sinaloa organization, one of the Mexican cartels most heavily involved in fentanyl trafficking, supposedly ordered its members to cease dealing fentanyl or face death. The Sinaloa leadership's statements against fentanyl, however, could be more publicity stunt than lasting change. Through 2023, the DEA detected no shortage of supply coming into the country, although reports in 2024 indicate the supply may be decreasing. One way for the government to target the fentanyl supply is to continue enhancing efforts to stop the supply of the precursor chemicals coming in from China that the cartels use to manufacture fentanyl. With fewer chemicals available, the cartels might be forced to further dilute the fentanyl by mixing it with less-lethal additives (such as xylazine), which would make the supply safer. This should be the first goal of any law enforcement strategy.

Safe supply is growing concept that has shown some success in Canada. In these programs, people with OUD who are judged at high risk of fatal overdose and for whom traditional drug treatment has not been suitable are prescribed medical hydromorphone (Dilaudid). Instead of playing Russian roulette with the dangerous and unpredictable street supply of fentanyl, they receive reliable doses of pharmaceutical-grade drugs under a health practitioner's care. Such programs have reduced overdoses and deaths and increased participation in the health care system. Unthinkable to many traditionalists, these programs may be the next step in the uphill battle to curb the rising deaths from our poisoned street drug supply. But isn't providing people with legitimately manufactured prescription pills just going back to the early days of the crisis when so many died? Yes, many people died, but not nearly as many who are dying from street fentanyl. Overdose deaths are five times higher today than they were in 2001. Much of the early crisis was caused by overprescribing and then suddenly cutting people off without tapering them down. We have adopted safeguards against overprescribing and physicians are more aware of the dangers of not properly tapering people off opioids. The deaths are catastrophically higher today not because of current prescribing but because the drug supply is toxic. People are being poisoned. If you had a daughter who was addicted to fentanyl, would you rather have her buying her drugs in an alley and shooting up behind a dumpster or getting her safe supply from a government-regulated health center and using in front of a health care provider who could talk to her about getting help? Safe supply will save lives.

Many individuals and organizations have proposed that decriminalizing street drugs is the best way to ensure safe supply. The World Health Organization has called for decriminalization of street drugs. The United Nations Development Programme has stated, "Laws criminalizing drug use/possession of small amounts of drugs for personal use impede the access of people who use drugs to basic services, such as housing, education, health care, employment, social protection, and treatment." Decriminalization means that people are allowed to have a small, specified amount of drugs for personal use. In some countries that have implemented decriminalization, those in possession of the legal amount can be civilly sanctioned or directed to treatment; in other countries, there are no penalties at all. People can be charged criminally, however, if they sell drugs or have more than the allowed amount.

In Portugal, which had high rates of drug usage, decriminalization has led to decreased crime, overdose deaths, and cases of HIV, as well as increased access to treatment. The prison population has gone down. Police focus on organized crime instead of street-level dealers.

The state of Oregon decriminalized drug use in 2021 following a 2020 ballot initiative, which also directed money raised from state marijuana sales to go toward increased treatment. The decriminalization occurred simultaneously with the arrival of fentanyl in Oregon as well as an unprecedented increase in homelessness. Opponents blamed the law, which was later overturned, for the increased deaths and the homelessness, not considering the impact of a drug supply now poisoned by fentanyl.

Homelessness is caused by a lack of affordable housing. People who lose their jobs due to addiction often can no longer afford high housing costs. A state like West Virginia that has high rates of drug use has not experienced homelessness on the scale Oregon has because housing costs are so low there. San Francisco, which has not decriminalized drug use, has similar problems to Oregon with homelessness and open drug use. To solve the drug crisis, we need to solve social problems like homelessness and poverty. If you are homeless and hungry and worried for your own personal safety, it may be hard to break free from addiction, particularly if you have no address, no phone, and nowhere to maintain your cleanliness. It is not easy to find legitimate employment in those circumstances. Some cities have turned to Houston, Texas, as an example of how to do housing right. There, nonprofits work in unison to help people with the single goal of getting them off the streets, and they are having success, partially thanks to less-restrictive building regulations than most cities.

The Oregon law didn't kick anyone out of their homes. It simply changed the penalties for simple possession from a misdemeanor (that could result in up to a year in jail) into a $100 fine that could be deferred if the person underwent a health assessment, which might include a referral to drug treatment. Most agree that the state has been slow to deliver on its promise of increased treatment. Others feel that treatment should be mandated, although most studies show that people mandated to treatment have much lower success rates than those who voluntarily enter treatment. Mandating people who are not ready for treatment may also deny limited beds to others who are ready for treatment. While decriminalization can lead to lower prison, court, and law enforcement costs, as well as enable people who might otherwise be in prison to continue to work and pay taxes, it does nothing to deal with the unsafe supply that is the primary cause of rising deaths.

Some people have called for complete legalization of drugs in the same manner we ended prohibition of alcohol. Indeed, the surest way to eliminate the unsafe street supply is to replace it with a regulated government safe supply. The primary difference between the opioids that pharmaceutical companies have made billions of profits on and the street opioids that have enriched the drug cartels is that the street opioids are of unpredictable strength and often contain other unknown and dangerous adulterants. When we prohibited alcohol in this country, the bootleg liquor sold on the streets poisoned countless Americans. Today we have a safe government-regulated alcohol supply as well as public consumption sites (bars, etc.). If we want to end the opioid deaths, particularly those deaths caused by fentanyl poisoning, we need to hold a conversation about legalization and government regulation of a safe supply.

I attended a forum of politicians in Hartford, including the governor, a US senator, a US representative, and the Hartford mayor, all good people who truly want to end this crisis. When I stood and told them it was time to consider decriminalization, legalization, safe injection sites, and safe supply, I could see them grimace. In our democracy, leaders only get to fight for their causes if they have the support of the people. They need their votes. This requires an educated populace. If people are not educated about the opioid epidemic, its causes, and the evidence behind positive solutions like increased medication-assisted treatment and harm reduction, they may be more likely to support funding for law enforcement to lock up drug users than pay for a space where "drug addicts" can freely use "illegal" drugs. A politician who advocates for a "safe injection site" is likely to face more voter disapproval than one who demands the "bad guys" be locked up. Come out strong for safe injection sites, and picture your opponent running an ad showing a grainy black-and-white scene of you walking around with "zombie junkies," then a quick cut to your opponent in full Technicolor with American flags in the background, shaking hands firmly with armed members of a police SWAT team. I have been at other forums where Connecticut Senator Richard Blumenthal, who has been an earnest listener to the people on the front lines and a great and appreciated advocate for harm reduction, has had to console parents of overdose victims, some who want blood vengeance against those who sold drugs to their child, while other parents who lost their children want to change the paradigm and focus on treatment instead of punishment. It is a hard wire to balance on. Harm reduction is one courageous stand, but for many, legalization would be five steps too far. It takes political courage, and it takes people who have built a career on integrity and who have the earned stature to tell voters that harm reduction is a smarter, more humane investment than building more prisons. Unfortunately, I do not think voters are ready for legalization and safe supply. Already, political ads have been run by some candidates warning of an apocalyptic future dominated by crime and fentanyl if their opponents are sent to office. No one is going to win control of Congress by promising free syringes and a warm place to shoot up, even if those hard-to-grasp concepts lead to less disease, fewer deaths, and more people getting into treatment so they can return to the lives they once had with their families and communities (including being contributing taxpayers to local, state, and federal treasuries).

But the choice is ours. Continue with the insanity of the drug war and its devastating effect on our citizenry, or recognize drug use as a disease and a public health issue and treat it accordingly, with empathy and evidence-based policy, not politics.

A Diamond

The landlord meets us outside on the avenue and leads us up the narrow stairs to the second-floor rooms. "She moved in five days ago," he says. "No one answers the door, and all my calls go to voicemail. I didn't want to go in without her permission." He unlocks the door for us. As soon as the door opens, I am hit with an unmistakable smell. "There's a body in there," I say.

The living room is devoid of furniture. She is in the bedroom, slumped forward in the frog position on the mattress. Her body is black and bloated. I can see the remnants of a foam cone around her mouth. The room is spare. Not even a TV. A half-unpacked suitcase. Some boxes. On the nightstand is a contact card from a battered women's shelter. Her ID shows a white woman in her thirties. In the photo, she looks skittish, uncertain of what may come next.

I try to imagine what her brief will say if her case is ever chosen for review by the fatality board. How did she start using? Did she have an accident? Was she pressured into using by an abusive spouse? What did she do for work? Did she have a family? Who were her friends? Did she have a mental illness? Had she ever been to rehab? To jail? What opportunities to help her were missed along the way?

Later that day her death will be entered into ODMAP—Overdose Detection Mapping Application Program—a national application that in 2022 tracked over 500,000 overdoses (fatal and nonfatal) nationwide. A red diamond indicating a fatal OD will appear on the street map of this Hartford neighborhood to mark her death, joining a thousand other diamonds on the map of Connecticut this year alone, and tens of thousands of diamonds on the nation's map.

Epilogue

My Brother's Keeper

Between June 2019 and May 2024, Connecticut EMS providers were required by law to report suspected opioid overdoses to the Connecticut Poison Control Center and answer a series of questions about the calls for surveillance purposes (age, gender, race, location of overdose, who gave the first naloxone, transport to the hospital, etc.), as well as providing a narrative. Beginning in June 2024, software was implemented to automatically download the electronic patient care reports for all suspected opioid overdoses. Part of my job has been to read those narratives and review and analyze the data. I have read over 20,000 reports to date. It is hard to convey the cumulative effect of reading these accounts. Each day I open the files, I read of death and despair. Parents do CPR on their children. Children do CPR on their parents. But more often I read the cases where solitary individuals are found lifeless and stiff—in an alley, under a bridge, or behind a locked bedroom door—too late for any intervention beyond covering

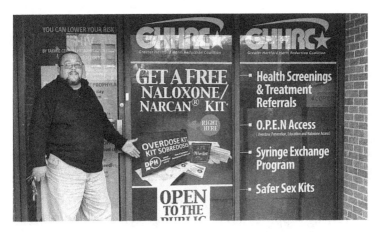

Mark Jenkins, harm reduction champion

their bodies with a sheet and calling the time. What is clear from these narratives is if a person is found quickly enough, the death is averted. I am cheered with each passing year as the number of bystander interventions increases, not just friends administering naloxone to each other but also strangers coming upon an overdosed person, taking naloxone out of their backpacks or purses, and saving a life. In 2019, 16 percent of all overdose users for whom 911 was called received bystander naloxone. In March 2024, the percentage was a record 32 percent. More people received naloxone from bystanders than responding fire departments.

Until we can make the structural changes necessary to expand treatment, end stigma, and right the social ills that fuel the epidemic, we need to continue to get as much naloxone as possible out on the street. I helped write a protocol for our naloxone leave-behind program, where EMS in our state can now leave naloxone kits with family and friends following overdoses. Such programs are spreading throughout the country as EMS embraces its role in providing harm reduction services.

I believe the growing availability of naloxone, the hard work of harm reductionists, the increasing availability of methadone and buprenorphine, as well as a slightly less toxic drug supply as dealers add more xylazine and decrease the amounts of fentanyl in their product are all contributing to the decline in overdose deaths we are now seeing nationwide. Connecticut, according to the CDC, reached its 12-month rolling high in fatal overdoses in November of 2021, the United States reached it's 12-month high in August of 2023. While promising the death toll is still far too high for anyone to ease off efforts, especially since almost all of these deaths are preventable. Let us pray that the declines continue and are lasting, rather than a pause onto a road higher. I hope we have learned our lessons.

When I am working 911, I look out for some of the friends I have made over the years—people who use drugs and have shared their stories, not only of how they got started but also of their struggles to get their lives together. Two such people are Kelley and Tom, whom I have known for nearly a decade now and whom I wrote about extensively in my book *Killing Season*. They returned to using drugs from a period of abstinence while living in New Jersey. They fell back into the life, living in an abandoned shed by the railroad tracks and occasionally working by packaging for a drug dealer. I see Tom one day after not seeing him for a month, and he looks well and strong. He says he has been painting houses and doing construction work, saving money. Kelley is in rehab and when she gets out, she is hoping to get a waitressing job. They have a promise of a place of their own in an apartment complex in the suburb where Tom has been doing some work. It is not the first time they have planned to leave the life, but I am hopeful this time will work for them. (Update: Kelley is out and on methadone and attending therapy sessions. She looks great!)

Another friend I wrote about is Veronica. I have not seen her in several years. When I review the EMS narratives, I always fear I will find her name attached to one. I am leaving Hartford Hospital one afternoon when I see a person get off the first bus at the corner ahead. It's Veronica! I have my partner pull to the curb. I get out and give her a big hug. She looks great. She tells me she has not used in over a year, and she just attended her daughter's wedding. She, too, is on medication-assisted treatment.

These three and many others helped me see the humanity of people who use drugs, a humanity I had been blinded to. I think of them as I work with Mark Jenkins and other advocates on the Connecticut Harm Reduction Alliance to fight for a more humane and more sensible drug policy. I stop in at The Drop on Albany Avenue and chat with the people there doing the front-line work of harm reduction. I am honored to be in their presence.

There is a little-known passage in the Hippocratic oath that I particularly like and that has become my creed: "Into whatsoever house I enter, I will enter to help the sick."

I hope that others will join me in our cause. Love and empathy for our neighbor will help us end this great scourge. We are all brothers and sisters on this earth. Let's be kind to each other.

Peace to all.

And carry naloxone.

Change

New Year's Eve. Overdose on the avenue—a woman in a tattered hoodie and black winter coat lies on the sidewalk next to a streetlight, with bystanders surrounding her. The woman, who looks to be in her forties, was talking to them when she slowly collapsed against the pole and then to the ground. If I stimulate her, she breathes, opens her eyes, and emits a high-pitched wail. Leave her be, and she stops breathing, her mouth open. I stimulate her again and then again. Her pupils are pinpoint, her oxygen saturation is in the 90s when I am stimulating her, and I can hear the ambulance sirens coming up the street. I am thinking I will get her in the ambulance, and if she keeps going apneic, I will put in an IV and give her just a tiny amount of naloxone, not even enough to rouse her but just enough to help her keep breathing on her own.

The local hospitals are seeing a record number of patients, the rooms are full, and the hallways are filled, even the back hallways, where they've never put patients before. They don't have staff to sit and monitor a heroin user's breathing. They'll dose her good with naloxone to wake her all the way up, even if it makes her sick.

When the ambulance arrives, we pick her up, and she opens her eyes and makes that high-pitched wail again. But as soon as the ambulance doors are closed, she goes apneic again. I nudge her a few times while I put in an IV, and then I mix the naloxone. I squirt 1 cc of saline from a 10 cc prefilled syringe, add 1 mg of naloxone to it, shake it to mix it, and then push 1 cc (0.1 mg of naloxone) through the hep-lock I put in her hand. Her breathing slowly picks up. Her eyes open, and she looks at me and swears softly.

"You are not in trouble," I say. "You overdosed. You weren't breathing adequately. I had to give you a tiny bit of naloxone."

She swears again. "I want to stop this," she says. "I need help. I want to enjoy my grandkids. I can't be doing this anymore."

I ask her if she has ever tried Suboxone. She says no. They have a program at the hospital, I tell her. They can get you on it. It works for some people. We can talk to them about getting you on it.

"I want to see my grandkids," she says.

The line at the hospital is several stretchers deep. My patient sings a gospel song while we wait for our assigned space.

"I was booooorn by the river."

She is not the greatest singer, and her lyrics are sporadic, but no one comes over to quiet her down. Her singing just adds to the din of the place. It is not uncommon for patients to break out into song while in the ED.

"Chaaaaange is gonna come, my brotha."

We end up putting her in a bed in the back hall. It takes me 10 minutes to find a nurse to give a report to. Her assigned nurse is in another room helping a doctor with an intubation. One of the other nurses in the pod went home sick, and they haven't been able to get anyone else to come in. I make my report brief. Fentanyl overdose, 0.1 naloxone IV, interested in getting on Suboxone. Got it, the nurse says, writing it down on a paper towel. I'll be sure and tell her. I stop back and tell the patient someone will be with her in a bit. She thanks me and goes back to singing, gesturing her arms as if to embrace the world.

"I will carry on, oh, yes, I will."

When I get back to the hospital several hours later, I check on her. She is gone, and no one can tell me if she left against medical advice or was seen and discharged. I don't know if anyone talked to her about Suboxone.

The sun has gone down. I have a few more hours left to go in my shift, the last of a long year.

PART THREE

Action

Key Points

10 Lessons from This Book

1. Opioids kill by stopping breathing.
2. Pinpoint pupils, depressed consciousness and depressed respirations are the hallmarks of an opioid overdose.
3. Opioid overdose deaths are preventable when the overdose is quickly recognized and naloxone is administered.
4. If you use opioids or have a family member or friend who does, you should have naloxone in your home and carry it with you; after administering naloxone, call 911.
5. Addiction is a chronic brain disease, not a crime.
6. Addiction is caused by a multiplicity of factors, including genetics and environmental influences.
7. Despite 50 years of the War on Drugs and trillions spent, drugs are cheaper, more readily available, and far more lethal today than they have ever been.
8. Fentanyl, which is 50 times stronger than heroin, is difficult for drug dealers to mix in predictable doses;

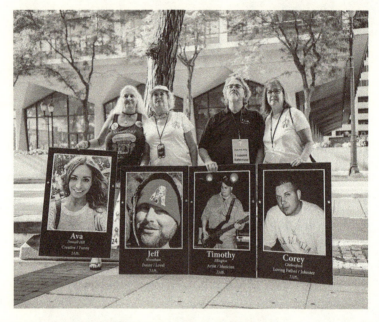

Today I Matter family members in Philadelphia

people die because they are unable to judge their drug's potency.
9. Most people who die of overdoses die using alone.
10. Harm reduction helps mitigate the harmful consequences of drug use; it keeps people alive until they are ready for change.
11. Medication-assisted treatment with methadone or buprenorphine is the gold standard of drug treatment.
12. Stigma kills.

Action Plan

A Seven-Point Agenda to Address the Crisis

According to the CDC, 101,168 Americans died of overdose in the 12-month period ending in April 2024, a 10 percent decrease from the previous year's record. Fentanyl continues to claim responsibility for most deaths, representing 92 percent of all opioid deaths in 2023. While the decline is a positive sign that harm reduction efforts, particularly increases in naloxone availability, may be having an impact, our citizens will continue to die as long as illicit fentanyl remains predominate in the nation's drug supply.

To prevent fentanyl deaths, we must take the following steps:

1. End the War on Drugs and the war on people who use drugs.
2. Recognize the drug use disorder as a public health problem, not a criminal one.

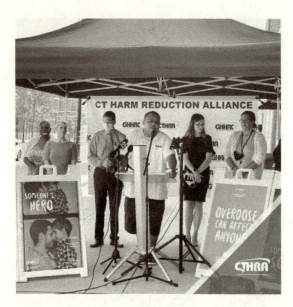

Harm reduction advocates

3. Reallocate funding to harm reduction and medical treatment, including offering Suboxone or methadone to all who meet the conditions.
4. Create a safe supply alternative by legalizing possession of small amounts of opioids and authorizing the production and regulation of pharmaceutical-grade heroin and/or fentanyl for users enrolled in public health programs.
5. Establish overdose prevention centers where users can use under the watch of a trained worker who has

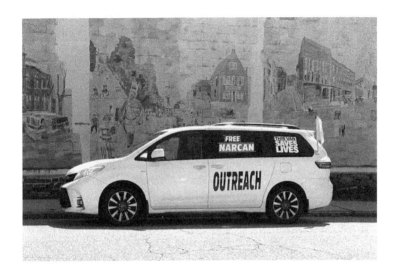

naloxone at hand, can refer patients to treatment, and can advise of safe-use practices and access to social services.
6. Create and support safe-use-alone applications to allow monitoring and rescue of patients who overdose when using alone.
7. Make naloxone available at little or no cost to the public.

If we are serious about stopping the deaths, we need to change our failed approaches of the past. Organize! Collaborate! Speak out!

ACKNOWLEDGMENTS

I am very fortunate that my work as a paramedic for American Medical Response in Hartford, Connecticut, and as the EMS coordinator at UConn John Dempsey Hospital has provided me with the opportunity not only to view the opioid crisis on the street level but to actively participate on state and local task forces and committees dealing with the crisis on a system level. I would like to thank my friend Dr. Richard Kamin, the Emergency Medical Services (EMS) medical director at UConn John Dempsey Hospital and the EMS medical director for the state of Connecticut, who recognized the important role EMS can play in battling the opioid epidemic and gave me the time to work on the EMS response. Thanks to Ralf Calciano, director of the state Office of Emergency Medical Services (OEMS), as well as Kitty Hickcox, Shauna Pangilinan, and Susan Logan at the state Department of Public Health, and Ramona Anderson at the Department of Mental Health and Addiction Services, for their commitment to the fight.

Brandon Bartell, Jeremy Dumas, and Jennifer Webb at American Medical Response have been strong advocates for patients with substance use issues and using the resources of ambulance services not only to treat patients in distress but to try to provide outreach and follow up. Thanks to Erica Robinson, Jerry Sneed, and all my other ambulance partners who make it worth going to work and who make me proud of the profession.

Thanks also to Robert Lawlor and Anna Gasinski at the New England High Intensity Drug Trafficking Area (HIDTA) program for the great job they do in Connecticut in providing resources and technical assistance. I would also like to thank Dr. Steve Wolf of the Connecticut Department of Consumer Protection, Dr. Robert Heimer of the Yale Public School of Health, and Bruce Baxter of New Britain Emergency Medical Services for their work and insights into the crisis. Thanks also to all my fellow committee members on the Statewide Harm Reduction Partnership (SHArP), especially Liz Evans and Cameron Breen, the Hartford Opioid Task Force, and the state Overdose Fatality Review Board.

Great thanks to Mark Jenkins and all those at the Greater Hartford Harm Reduction Coalition (now the Connecticut Harm Reduction Alliance [CHRA]) for all they have taught me over the years. Mike Grace, Alixe Ditmore, Alex Diaz, Brian Sawyer, Jose Lozado, Michael Morris, Chris Ortiz, River Rose, Courtney Dollar, and all who work with CHRA are true heroes in this fight. Special thanks to Andrea McNight for the kindness she showed my daughter, Zoey, when Zoey volunteered at CHRA's the Drop.

Thanks to John Lalley and Richard Mogensen and other parents for sharing their stories of their children's lives and their losses. John runs the foundation Today I Matter (https://www.todayimatter.org/about.html) in honor of his son, Tim. Richard is the author of *Cody's Story: A Son's Death and A Father's Battle Against Opioids*.

Thanks to the late former US senator and governor of Connecticut, Lowell P. Weicker, for fighting for those without access to power and for current US Senator Richard Blumenthal for continuing the fight. Thanks to Connecticut State Senator Saud Anwar for his leadership in the state.

I would like to thank my intrepid agent, Jane Dystel, for her support over the years and Robin Coleman for encouraging me to write this book and for shepherding it through the process at Johns Hopkins University Press. Thanks to all those who contributed so much to its production.

Finally, and most importantly, thanks to my patients over the years who shared their stories with me and helped me understand the complexity of the epidemic and see the humanity in all.

GLOSSARY

abstinence. Not currently using drugs; abstaining from drug use.

addict. A stigmatizing word that dehumanizes a person by judging them by their behavior. The preferred term is *person with substance use disorder*.

addiction. A chronic, relapsing brain disease and not a character flaw. People who become addicted experience chemical changes in their brain's reward system that produce compulsion, making it difficult to exert self-control and often causing them to act against their own best interests. It is believed that genetics account for 50 percent of a person's risk for developing addiction, with environmental and developmental factors accounting for the rest. Drug addiction can be successfully treated, but since it is a chronic, not an acute, disease, relapse is not unexpected.

benzodiazepines. Central nervous system depressants that are used to treat anxiety, seizures, and depression. They include Ativan (lorazepam), Diazepam (Valium), Alprazolam (Xanax), and **Clonazepam (Klonopin)**. Combining them with opioids is dangerous and can lead to overdose and death if taken in sufficient quantities.

bioavailability. The percentage of a drug that is actively used by the body. Drugs injected intravenously have a higher bioavailability than those ingested orally.

buprenorphine. An FDA-approved opioid that is used to treat substance use disorder. It helps reduce cravings and does not produce the type of euphoria caused by heroin or fentanyl. It comes in a pill or sublingual film and needs to be taken daily.

carfentanil. A synthetic opioid that is used primarily to tranquilize large animals, such as elephants. It is purportedly 100 times stronger than fentanyl. It was attributed to a rise in deaths in several states, such as Ohio and Pennsylvania, around 2017 before declining. The decline has been attributed to increased regulation of the drug's sources in China, but others believe the potency of the drug made it too hard to successfully blend into the drug supply without killing too many people.

chronic pain. Over 100 million Americans suffer from chronic pain. The overprescription of opioids pushed many into addiction. The subsequent backlash against opioid prescriptions has upset some people who are no longer able to get opioids or sufficient opioids for their pain. Some of them have been forced to turn to far more dangerous street drugs. Doctors have to walk a fine line with their patients to treat their pain without exposing those prone to addiction to opioid's dangers. More consideration is now given to nonopioid pain medications and other pain treatment methods.

"clean" and "dirty." Stigmatizing terms that are often used to compare someone who is not currently using drugs ("clean") with someone who is currently using drugs ("dirty").

cocaine. A highly addictive stimulant that causes intense euphoria. It comes as a white powder that can be snorted or injected or in small rock form called crack that can be smoked by heating it and inhaling the fumes.

comorbidity. The co-occurrence of two disorders, such as substance use disorder and mental health disorder.

COVID and the opioid crisis. The COVID pandemic and its lockdowns coincided with a rise in overdose deaths during that period. Established drug supply lines experienced disruptions that forced users to buy from unfamiliar sources, increasing their chances of overdosing. Training and substance outreach programs were either closed or had limited hours. Some moved online, which worked for those who had a home and a computer but not for those who were displaced. People had less access to the help they needed as well as reduced access to naloxone and clean needles. Isolating people with existing mental health issues may have led former users (with now lowered tolerance) to return to substance use. The increased release of prisoners with a history of drug use put them at risk for overdose due to their lack of tolerance. Patients with undiagnosed COVID-19 may have been less resilient if they did overdose due to reduced respiratory capacity. People without work, with increased economic and social pressures, may have sought escape. And probably most likely of all, more people used alone, with no one there to administer naloxone in case of overdose.

decriminalization. Removes criminal penalties for illegal possession and personal drug use. Under decriminalization, drugs may still be illegal, but the punishments may include referral to services or small fines. Decriminalization focuses on health and enables law enforcement to save its resources for pursuing major drug trafficking organizations instead of street users. It frees up prison space, helps prevent people from hiding their drug use and overdosing alone, and may encourage people to seek treatment without fear of being incarcerated or stigmatized. Decriminalization should be implemented hand in hand with harm reduction and sufficient treatment services. Many states have decriminalized marijuana. Oregon decriminalized all drugs in 2020, but that was subsequently rolled back in 2024.

dependence. When someone feels they cannot function without a certain drug. Dependence can be physical or psychological.

detoxification. Cleaning the body of drugs or alcohol. This can be accomplished either by going cold turkey through unaided withdrawal, which is considered dangerous, or assisted with medications to ease the symptoms of withdrawal.

drug courts. These courts offer an alternative to jail by sending some people to treatment instead of locking them up. Participants are required to be abstinent and can be punished for relapsing. There is some controversy over their effect on recidivism as well as their cost. They still treat substance use as a crime and punish those who relapse, an often-anticipated part of recovery.

fentanyl. A synthetic addictive opioid 50 times more powerful than heroin that has largely come to replace heroin throughout much of the United States. Its potency makes it difficult for dealers to produce reliable doses. It is also the active ingredient in many counterfeit pills sold as prescription pills, such as Percocet, oxycodone, and Xanax. Fentanyl represents the third and most deadly wave of the current opioid epidemic. Fentanyl produced by pharmaceutical companies is commonly used in the United States for pain relief, including as specially formulated skin patches to provide time-release pain relief.

harm reduction. According to the National Harm Reduction Coalition, "A set of practical strategies and ideas aimed at reducing negative consequences associated with drug use. Harm Reduction is also a movement for social justice built on a belief in, and respect for, the rights of people who use drugs." Harm reduction includes community naloxone, syringe exchange, street drug testing, and overdose prevention centers.

heroin. An illegal addictive opioid produced from the poppy plant that has long been misused. Heroin represents the second wave of the opioid overdose crisis. Heroin deaths began rising in the United States in 2010 with the introduction of a tamper-proof oxycodone, causing many pill users to switch to the cheaper and more readily available heroin. Heroin does have a legal medicinal use in Great Britain but not in the United States.

iron law of prohibition. A theory proposed by the drug activist Richard Cowan that states, "As law enforcement becomes more intense, the potency of prohibited substances increases." This was true during prohibition as hard liquor was easier to smuggle and more profitable than bootleg beer, and it is certainly true in the opioid crisis as fentanyl, 50 times stronger than heroin, has almost entirely replaced heroin due to ease of trafficking and higher profits.

junkie. A stigmatizing name for drug users that came from a view of drug users searching through trash, or "junk," for food or items to sell. These people became known as junkies, human trash.

legalization. The act of making drug use and possession of drugs legal and not punishable by law enforcement. Ideally the drug supply is regulated and taxed by the government to ensure consistent quality.

medication-assisted treatment (MAT). Medications such as buprenorphine, methadone, and naltrexone used to treat opioid use disorders in conjunction with counseling and behavioral therapy.

medications for opioid use disorder (MOUD). *See* medication-assisted treatment (MAT).

methadone. An FDA-approved long-acting opioid that has been shown to be effective in helping people get off stronger opioids, such as heroin and fentanyl. Methadone reduces cravings without producing the great euphoria of other opioids. Many people are on methadone long term. It is usually administered in a liquid form at a clinic where participants are expected to go each day for their dose.

methamphetamine. An illicit short-acting stimulant that produces great euphoria. Many opioid users are also addicted to methamphetamine, which they use to counter the sedative effect of opioids. Methamphetamine is the drug trafficked in the TV series *Breaking Bad*.

morphine. An opioid distilled from opium. Originally, it was marketed as a cure for opium addiction and sold over the counter. People soon became addicted to it. Morphine is commonly used in our health care system as a prescription for pain relief.

naloxone. An FDA-approved opioid antagonist. Naloxone knocks opioids off the brain receptors that control breathing, effectively reversing opioid overdoses if given in time. It can be administered by professionals and laypeople. In 2023, intranasal naloxone was approved for over-the-counter sales. Anyone who uses opioids or has a close friend or family member who uses opioids should have naloxone available in case of an overdose.

Naltrexone. A medication used to treat opioid use disorder, commonly given as a four-week shot. Naltrexone blocks the euphoric and sedative effects of opioids but does nothing to curb cravings.

Narcan. The brand name for a popular form of intranasal naloxone. It is often used interchangeably with the generic naloxone to describe any use of the drug.

opiate. A drug naturally derived from opium, the poppy plant. This includes morphine and heroin. Opiates are opioids.

opioid. A type of drug that acts on the opioid receptors in the brain to provide analgesia (pain relief). The class includes natural opiates and synthetic drugs. Common prescription opioids include buprenorphine, codeine, fentanyl, hydrocodone, hydrocodone and acetaminophen (Vicodin), hydromorphone (Dilaudid), meperidine (Demerol), methadone, morphine, oxycodone (OxyContin), oxycodone and acetaminophen (Percocet), and tramadol (Ultram). Illicit opioids include heroin, fentanyl, and carfentanil. Opioids are known to be addictive and when taken in sufficient quantities can lead to overdose and death by depressing or stopping breathing. Cessation of use in those addicted can produce unpleasant withdrawal symptoms.

oxycodone. An addictive prescription pill used to treat pain.

OxyContin. A time-released version of oxycodone that was first marketed by Purdue Pharma in 1995. Their aggressive marketing that downplayed its addictive qualities is credited with launching the first wave of the opioid epidemic.

potency. The amount of a drug needed to produce a given effect. Drugs produced by American pharmaceutical laboratories have a reliable potency. Illicit street drugs mixed by drug dealers have wildly varying potencies that make it difficult for users to gauge the drug's effect on them and easy to overdose.

Purdue Pharma. The manufacturer of OxyContin. They have been sued for billions of dollars for their false advertising and aggressive marketing of the drug despite knowing its dangers.

racial disparities in the opioid crisis. Population data shows increasing disparities between certain racial groups in the overdose crisis. Currently the death rate among Black Americans is increasing precipitously, while treatment options remain fewer than those available to other groups.

recovery coach/peer support. A person from a community organization with a history of drug use (lived experience) who is in recovery and assists other people who have recently overdosed in navigating the avenues of recovery. They may meet them in the ED and then follow them afterward, helping them find the help they need.

relapse. A recurrence of a past condition. In substance use terms, a person relapses when they start using drugs again after a period of recovery.

routes of exposure. The various forms in which drugs are taken. Opioids can be swallowed in pill or liquid form. They can be snorted as powder. They can be inhaled as vapor through smoking. (In this method, which is particularly used with black tar heroin—most common in the western United States—the heroin is placed on foil, and a heat source is applied underneath. Users inhale the vapor.) Opioids can be injected into a vein, into a muscle, or under the skin. They can also be absorbed through the skin using a special formulated patch. Finally, in a process known as "boofing," they can be inserted into the rectum to be absorbed into the gastrointestinal tract.

safe injection site. A place where people can use drugs in a clean, safe environment under the watchful eyes of harm reduction health personnel. Insite in Vancouver is the model. Since opening in 2003 as the first safe injection site in North America, they have had over 4 million uses, over 11,000 overdoses reversed, and not a single death. In the United States, there are two safe injection sites in New York City, as well as many unofficial sites. These sites are also called overdose prevention centers and safe consumption sites. The 3rd U.S. Circuit Court of Appeals court ruled that such sites are illegal under the crack house statutes, but as of the end of 2024, no federal action has been taken to close these sites.

stigma. A mark of shame synonymous with disgrace, dishonor, ignominy, and humiliation. The stigma of being an "addict" implies that the addict is to blame for their actions. It not only suggests moral judgment against a person, but it also inspires fear in others and isolates and discriminates. The stigmatized become stereotypes, not people.

suboxone. A medication used to treat opioid use disorder; it combines buprenorphine and naloxone. The naloxone is added to prevent users from injecting the buprenorphine in an attempt to get high. Suboxone taken the prescribed route, sublingually, relieves cravings without producing the highs typical of heroin or fentanyl.

substance use disorder. According to the National Institute of Mental Health, substance use disorder is "a treatable mental disorder that affects a person's brain and behavior, leading to their inability to control their use of substances like legal or illegal drugs, alcohol, or medications."

syringe exchange. Syringe service exchange programs (SSPs) provide people who use drugs with clean needles and syringes, help dispose of used equipment, and provide access to treatment and other needed social services. They have been credited with helping reduce the transmission of diseases such as AIDS and hepatitis C, as well as helping get many people into drug treatment.

tolerance. When someone uses a drug for a period of time, their body adapts to it, and they require more of the drug to achieve the effect they had on initial use. Conversely, if they stop using a drug, their tolerance goes down and they can overdose if they use the same amount they used when they were using regularly.

triggers. Stimuli that cause people who once used drugs to feel the urge to use drugs again. A trigger may be a place, a friend, an emotion, or even a song that triggers a memory associated with past drug use.

twelve-step program. A form of substance use treatment modeled after Alcoholics Anonymous, where members admit their powerlessness to control their drug use that has become unmanageable, give themselves up to a higher power, work with a sponsor to examine the errors they have made and the people they have hurt, and work to make amends and help others.

War on Drugs. In 1971, President Richard Nixon started America's War on Drugs that continues today. The war led to mass incarceration, cost trillions of dollars, and had little to show in terms of results, as the drug problem in America today is killing more than it ever has. In 2018, law enforcement agencies in the United States made over 1.65 million drug arrests. That's one drug arrest every 19 seconds. The demand and supply of drugs remains as high as ever and the potency of drugs stronger and far more lethal than ever.

withdrawal. Symptoms such as nausea, vomiting, and pain that develop when a person who is dependent on a drug stops using that drug. Opioid withdrawal is particularly painful and has been described as having the worst flu times a million. The symptoms make it difficult for someone to rid their system of drugs as they can relieve the symptoms simply by using drugs again.

Xylazine. An animal tranquilizer that drug dealers add to their fentanyl mixture. Because fentanyl ebbs within three to four hours or sooner, adding xylazine adds "legs" to the drug, meaning the person's high lasts longer. Xylazine can cause severe skin necrosis not only when injected but also when snorted or smoked. It is also known as "tranq."

A NOTE ON SOURCES

Introduction

Throughout this book, I cite various death statistics. This information comes from federal sources (e.g., Centers for Disease Control and Prevention) and state sources (e.g, the Connecticut Office of the Chief Medical Examiner). See, for example, Merianne Rose Spencer, Matthew Garnett, and Arialdi M. Miniño, "Drug Overdose Deaths in the United States, 2002–2022," Centers for Disease Control and Prevention, December 26, 2023, https://doi.org/10.15620/cdc:135849; Connecticut Office of the Chief Medical Examiner, "Connecticut Accidental Drug Intoxication Deaths," Office of the Chief Medical Examiner, March 1, 2024, https://portal.ct.gov/-/media/OCME/Statistics/Calendar-Years.pdf.

The increase in fatal overdoses is outpacing the increase in illicit drug use. This report shows decreasing opioid and fentanyl abuse: Substance Abuse and Mental Health Services Administration, *2023 Companion Infographic Report: Results from the 2021, 2022, and 2023: National Surveys on Drug Use and Health* (Substance Abuse and Mental Health Services Administration, 2024), https://www.samhsa.gov/data/sites/default/files/reports/rpt47096/2023-nsduh-companion-report.pdf.

The information about fentanyl's potency and what amount constitutes a lethal dose of fentanyl comes from the Drug Enforcement Administration. Just 2 mg of fentanyl is a tiny amount—equal to about 10 grains of table salt. Some people who use fentanyl regularly may be able to tolerate much more, but for an opioid-naïve person, ten grains could be enough to stop their breathing and cause death if the overdose is not quickly recognized and treated with naloxone. Typically, fentanyl is mixed with cutting agents, so determining just how many milligrams of fentanyl are in a $2 wax fold of white powder or in a small counterfeit pill is impossible for anyone without access to sophisticated laboratory testing equipment. See US Drug Enforcement Administration, "Facts About Fentanyl," DEA, n.d., https://www.dea.gov/resources/facts-about-fentanyl.

Just how many American struggle with drug addiction is hard to know. I encountered widely varying numbers. The data here comes from the National Center for Drug Abuse Statistics (NCDAS) and the Substance Abuse and Mental Health Services Administration (SAMHSA): Jaleesa Bustamante, "Drug Abuse Statistics," NCDAS, January 1, 2023, https://drugabusestatistics.org/; Douglas Richesson, Iva Magas, Samantha Brown, and Jennifer M. Hoenig, *Key Substance Use and Mental Health Indicators in the United States: Results from the 2022 National Survey on Drug Use and Health* (Center for Behavioral Health Statistics and Quality, Substance Abuse and Mental Health Services Administration, 2023), https://www.samhsa.gov/data/sites/default/files/reports/rpt42731/2022-nsduh-nnr.pdf.

Chapter 1

Many Americans know someone who has died of an overdose. These deaths have a powerful impact on our society, as described in this *American Journal of Public Health* article: Alison Athey, Beau Kilmer, and Julie Cerel, "An Overlooked Emergency: More Than One in Eight US Adults Have Had Their Lives Disrupted by Drug Overdose Deaths," *American Journal of Public Health* 114, no. 3 (March 1, 2024): 276–79, https://doi.org/10.2105/ajph.2023.307550.

Getting a simple prescription for an opioid from a trusted doctor carries risks that most patients are unaware of. It is hard to believe that some can develop an elevated risk for attachment to opioids in as few as five days of use, as described in this research paper: Anuj Shah, Corey J. Hayes, and Bradley C. Martin, "Characteristics of Initial Prescription Episodes and Likelihood of Long-Term Opioid Use—United States, 2006–2015," *Morbidity and Mortality Weekly Report* 66, no. 10 (March 17, 2017): 265–69, https://doi.org/10.15585/mmwr.mm6610a1.

These next three documents detail the pervasive numbers of opioid prescriptions in our country that are fortunately declining: Alan R. Roth and Andy Lazris, "Appropriate Use of Opioids for Chronic Pain," *American Family Physician* 102, no. 6 (September 15, 2020): 335–37, https://www.aafp.org/pubs/afp/issues/2020/0915/p335.pdf; National Center for Injury Prevention and Control, Division of Unintentional Injury Prevention, Centers for Disease Control and Prevention, "Opioid Painkiller Prescribing," *CDC Vital Signs*, July 2014, https://www.cdc.gov/vitalsigns/pdf/2014-07-vitalsigns.pdf; Centers for Disease Control and Prevention, "United States Dispensing Rate Maps," November 7, 2024, https://www.cdc.gov/overdose-prevention/data-research/facts-stats/us-dispensing-rate-maps.html.

Connecticut lawmakers have worked to safeguard prescribing by limiting the length of standard opioid prescriptions. See Department of Consumer Protection, "Connecticut Laws Impacting Prescribing and Practice," CT.gov, https://portal.ct.gov/DCP/Prescription-Monitoring-Program/Connecticut-Laws-Impacting-Prescribing-and-Practice.

This article details the risk of subsequent drug use by patients who were prescribed opioids at a young age: R. Miech, L. Johnston, P. M. O'Malley, K. M. Keyes, K. Heard, "Prescription Opioids in Adolescence and Future

Opioid Misuse," *Pediatrics* 136, no. 5 (November 2015): e1169–77, https://doi.org/10.1542/peds.2015-1364.

This article makes a convincing case that people with high adverse childhood experiences (ACEs) are at higher risk of later substance use and addiction: Myriam Forster, Amy L. Gower, Iris W. Borowsky, and Barbara J. McMorris, "Associations Between Adverse Childhood Experiences, Student-Teacher Relationships, and Non-medical Use of Prescription Medications Among Adolescents," *Addictive Behaviors* 68 (May 1, 2017): 30–34, https://doi.org/10.1016/j.addbeh.2017.01.004.

The CDC's State Unintentional Drug Overdose Reporting System (SUDORS) Dashboard provides fascinating insight into factors behind fatal overdoses, including percentage of fatal overdose patients who have had mental health issues and the number who had prior overdoses. The dashboard currently has information from 29 states and the District of Columbia. Each jurisdiction can be independently searched. See Centers for Disease Control and Prevention, "SUDORS Dashboard: Fatal Drug Overdose Data," December 12, 2024, https://www.cdc.gov/overdose-prevention/data-research/facts-stats/sudors-dashboard-fatal-overdose-data.html.

The science behind addiction is fascinating, as detailed in this paper about thrill-seeking and substance use: Reece Alvarez, "Thrill-Seeking and Substance Abuse: Common Link Found in Brain Anatomy," the Science Explorer, April 12, 2016, https://www.thescienceexplorer.com/thrill-seeking-and-substance-abuse-common-link-found-in-brain-anatomy-1397.

Genetics play a role in addiction. They are not a guarantee of drug misuse or addiction but rather a possible contributing factor. See Alexander S. Hatoum, Sarah M. C. Colbert, Emma C. Johnson, et al., "Multivariate

Genome-Wide Association Meta-Analysis of Over 1 Million Subjects Identifies Loci Underlying Multiple Substance Use Disorders," *Nature Mental Health* 1, no. 3 (March 22, 2023): 210–23, https://doi.org/10.1038/s44220-023-00034-y.

In this book, I often cite Connecticut statistics based on EMS calls that were tabulated through the state's unique opioid overdose reporting system that required EMS to call the Connecticut Poison Control Center following each suspected overdose they responded to. The data collected over five years gave fascinating insights into the opioid crisis. See Connecticut Department of Public Health, *Statewide Opioid Reporting Directive (SWORD) 2023 Annual Report* (Connecticut Department of Public Health, 2023), https://portal.ct.gov/-/media/departments-and-agencies/dph/dph/ems/pdf/sword/sword-newsletters/2023/sword-annual-report-2022-23final.pdf.

The Connecticut Office of the Child Advocate reviews child fatality cases. See Sarah Eagan and Office of the Child Advocate, *Child Fatality Investigation Findings & Recommendations* (State of Connecticut Office of the Child Advocate, 2024), https://portal.ct.gov/-/media/oca/oca-recent-publications/ocamarcellofatalityreviewfinalreport2024.pdf.

Overdose deaths among the elderly are often unrecognized and appear to be getting worse. See, for example, Holly Hedegaard, Arialdi M. Miniño, and Margaret Warner, "Drug Overdose Deaths in the United States, 2001–2021," Centers for Disease Control and Prevention, December 22, 2022, https://doi.org/10.15620/cdc:122556.

This excellent report published by the US Department of Health and Human Services details the occupations most at risk for opioid death: Rachael M. Billock, Andrea L. Steege, and Arialdi Miniño, "Drug Overdose Mortality by Usual Occupation and Industry: 46 U.S. States and New

York City, 2020," *National Vital Statistics Reports* 72, no. 7 (August 22, 2023), https://dx.doi.org/10.15620/cdc:128631.

As polypharmacy—the use of multiple drugs—increases, it is important to understand what each drug does and how they may interact. Fentanyl remains the deadliest cause of sudden overdose death. See S. Ahmed, Z. Sarfraz, and A. Sarfraz, "Editorial: A Changing Epidemic and the Rise of Opioid-Stimulant Co-Use," *Frontiers in Psychiatry* 13 (July 6, 2022): 918197, https://doi.org/10.3389/fpsyt.2022.918197; Enrique Rivero, "Overdose Deaths from Fentanyl Laced Stimulants Have Risen 50-Fold Since 2010," UCLA Health, September 13, 2023, https://www.uclahealth.org/news/overdose-deaths-fentanyl-laced-stimulants-have-risen-50-fold.

This article details the havoc long-term cocaine use wreaks on the body: K. Bachi, V. Mani, D. Jeyachandran, Z. A. Fayad, R. Z. Goldstein, and N. Alia-Klein, "Vascular Disease in Cocaine Addiction," *Atherosclerosis* 262 (July 2017): P154–62, https://doi.org/10.1016/j.atherosclerosis.2017.03.019.

Drugs have different bioavailability depending on their method of administration. See J. F. Jin, L. L. Zhu, M. Chen, et al., "The Optimal Choice of Medication Administration Route Regarding Intravenous, Intramuscular, and Subcutaneous Injection," *Patient Preference and Adherence* 2015, no. 9 (July 2, 2015): 923–42, https://doi.org/10.2147/PPA.S87271.

There is a stereotype that almost everyone who overdoses will overdose again and again. The data I discuss in this book shows this is not true. Still, if someone has overdosed once, they are at risk for a future overdose and deserve our help to avoid that end. See Scott G. Weiner, Olesya Baker, Dana Bernson, and Jeremiah D. Schuur, "One Year Mortality of Patients Treated with Naloxone for Opioid Overdose by Emergency Medical Services," *Substance Abuse* 43, no. 1 (2022): 99–103, https://doi.org/10.1080/08897077.2020.1748163.

The 91 percent figure of fatal overdose patients who had no previous recorded overdoses is from the CDC SUDORS dashboard previously mentioned: Centers for Disease Control and Prevention, "SUDORS Dashboard."

Chapter 2

Many years ago, I came across this saying from an old Boston paramedic, who to my knowledge is still nameless. He said people "take opiates and other sedatives specifically to induce a pleasant stupor. If they're lethargic and hard to arouse but still breathing effectively, it's not an overdose. It's a dose." Simply using opioids is not an emergency; it's when the opioids slow a person's breathing to the point that it impacts their brain and other organs that we need to act.

I have been on scenes where bystanders or first responders have treated people who were perfectly all right and on scenes where they have not recognized the person is not just sleeping but is starved for oxygen. It is also important to understand that an overdose doesn't always occur as soon as drugs are administered. It depends on many factors, including the route of administration, which can affect the amount of the drug the body can absorb and the onset of action. These two papers discuss the bioavailability of oxycodone through various routes: Rosemary Stevens and Salim M. Ghazi, "Routes of Opioid Analgesic Therapy in the Management of Cancer Pain," *Cancer Control* 7, no. 2 (March 1, 2000): 132–41, https://doi.org/10.1177/107327480000700203; M. R. Lofwall, D. E. Moody, W. B. Fang, P. A. Nuzzo, and S. L. Walsh, "Pharmacokinetics of Intranasal Crushed OxyContin and Intravenous Oxycodone in Nondependent Prescription Opioid Abusers," *Journal of Clinical Pharmacology* 52 no. 4 (April 2012): 600–606, https://doi.org/10.1177/0091270011401620.

Chapter 3

This is a link to the National Institute on Drug Abuse's naloxone DrugFacts page: "Naloxone DrugFacts," National Institute on Drug Abuse, February 12, 2024, https://nida.nih.gov/publications/drugfacts/naloxone.

Naloxone doesn't have to knock all the opioids off the receptor sites, just enough to restore breathing. No opioid has been found yet that does not respond to naloxone. This study is useful in understanding naloxone's effectiveness: J. Melichar, David Nutt, and Andrea L. Malizia, "Naloxone Displacement at Opioid Receptor Sites Measured in Vivo in the Human Brain," *European Journal of Pharmacology* 459, no. 2–3 (January 1, 2003): 217–19, https://doi.org/10.1016/s0014-2999(02)02872-8.

Connecticut EMS responders were required to call the state poison control center after each suspected opioid overdose and answer a series of questions, including who administered the first naloxone. The data was tracked for five years and identified many interesting trends, including the increasing number of naloxone administrations given by bystanders. See Connecticut Department of Public Health, *Statewide Opioid Reporting Directive (SWORD) 2023 Annual Report*.

The intranasal device that delivers naloxone is super easy to use as opposed to the older atomizer device. See P. Krieter, N. Chiang, S. Gyaw, et al., "Pharmacokinetic Properties and Human Use Characteristics of an FDA-Approved Intranasal Naloxone Product for the Treatment of Opioid Overdose," *Journal of Clinical Pharmacology* 56, no. 10 (2016):1243–53, https://doi.org/10.1002/jcph.759.

Too many people assume more is better. This study shows the drawbacks of higher-dose naloxone without increased benefits: Emily R. Payne, Sharon Stancliff, Kirsten Rowe, Jason A. Christie, and Michael W. Dailey,

"Comparison of Administration of 8-Milligram and 4-Milligram Intranasal Naloxone by Law Enforcement During Response to Suspected Opioid Overdose—New York, March 2022–August 2023," *Morbidity and Mortality Weekly Report* 73, no. 5 (February 8, 2024), https://www.cdc.gov/mmwr/volumes/73/wr/pdfs/mm7305a4-H.pdf.

For a good article describing the debate over naloxone dosing as the pharmaceutical companies try to promote new products, see Ellen Eldridge, "Stronger Opioid Overdose Reversal Medicines Worsen Patients' Withdrawal Symptoms," Now Habersham, updated January 2, 2024, https://nowhabersham.com/stronger-opioid-overdose-reversal-medicines-worsen-patients-withdrawal-symptoms/.

Naloxone does not raise the dead. It can revive the unconscious and the not breathing, but after a person's heart has stopped, cardiac drugs such as epinephrine are needed to restore circulation. See Cameron Dezfulian, Aaron M. Orkin, Bradley A. Maron, et al., "Opioid-Associated Out-of-Hospital Cardiac Arrest: Distinctive Clinical Features and Implications for Health Care and Public Responses: A Scientific Statement from the American Heart Association," *Circulation* 143, no. 16 (April 20, 2021), https://doi.org/10.1161/cir.0000000000000958.

Naloxone will only work on opioids, not on other classifications of drugs or alcohol, which many people ingest with opioids. If a person has used opioids, naloxone will help counteract the effects of the opioids in patients who have used other drugs but won't reverse the effects of the other drugs, which are usually less lethal. See "Other Drugs," Centers for Disease Control and Prevention, May 8, 2024, https://www.cdc.gov/overdose-prevention/about/polysubstance-overdose.html.

"I didn't take anything" is a common response from revived patients, as the CT SWORD data reveals. See Connecticut Department of Public

Health, "Patients Resuscitated with Naloxone Often Deny Drug Use," *CT EMS SWORD Statewide Opioid Reporting Directive Newsletter*, September 2023, https://portal.ct.gov/-/media/departments-and-agencies/dph/dph/ems/pdf/sword/sword-newsletters/2023/swordsept2023nl_approved.pdf.

The first priority is restoring breathing. Don't let possible side effects prevent you from treating someone. This article explains possible reasons for post-resuscitation dyspnea: Justin Kosirog and Wesley Eilbert, "Dyspnea After a Heroin Overdose," *Emergency Physicians Monthly*, February 7, 2018, https://epmonthly.com/article/dyspnea-heroin-overdose/.

The surgeon general's appeal to Americans to carry naloxone is found here: Office of the Surgeon General, "U.S. Surgeon General's Advisory on Naloxone and Opioid Overdose," HHS.gov, April 8, 2022, https://www.hhs.gov/surgeongeneral/reports-and-publications/addiction-and-substance-misuse/advisory-on-naloxone/index.html.

When people use alone at home, there is no one to find them and deliver naloxone. SWORD data reveals a high death toll in residences: Connecticut Department of Public Health, *Statewide Opioid Reporting Directive (SWORD) 2022 Annual Report* (Connecticut Department of Public Health, 2022), https://portal.ct.gov/-/media/departments-and-agencies/dph/dph/ems/pdf/sword/sword-newsletters/2022/2022-sword-annual-report---slides.pdf.

This interesting study showed that while naloxone may be over the counter, it is most often behind the counter: Jeffery Liu, Bianca Schutz, Skye Fredericks, Imani Hill, Gautam Chaudhry, and Katharine Neill Harris, "How Available Is Over-the-Counter Naloxone in Houston?" Baker Institute, February 2, 2024, https://www.bakerinstitute.org/research/how-available-over-counter-naloxone-houston.

Connecticut allows pharmacists to write prescriptions for naloxone. Now that naloxone is over the counter, the prescriptions can help defray the high over-the-counter cost for people with insurance, including Medicare and Medicaid. See "Naloxone Prescribing by Pharmacists," CT.gov. https://portal.ct.gov/dcp/drug-control-division/drug-control/naloxone-prescribing-by-pharmacists.

Naloxone continues to be effective after its labeled expiration date. See Center for Drug Evaluation and Research, "FDA Announces Shelf-Life Extension for Naloxone Nasal Spray," US Food and Drug Administration, January 17, 2024, https://www.fda.gov/drugs/drug-safety-and-availability/fda-announces-shelf-life-extension-naloxone-nasal-spray; S. Pruyn, J. Frey, B. Baker, et al, "Quality Assessment of Expired Naloxone Products from First-Responders' Supplies," *Prehospital Emergency Care* 23, no. 5 (2019): 647–53, https://doi.org/10.1080/10903127.2018.1563257.

This paper documents two case studies of people who self-administered naloxone: T. C. Green, M. Ray, S. E. Bowman, M. McKenzie, and J. D. Rich, "Two Cases of Intranasal Naloxone Self-Administration in Opioid Overdose," *Substance Abuse* 35, no. 2 (2014): 129–32, https://doi.org/10.1080/08897077.2013.825691.

Good Samaritan laws have been effective, as discussed in this GAO report: United States Government Accountability Office, "Drug Misuse: Most States Have Good Samaritan Laws and Research Indicates They May Have Positive Effects," Report to Congressional Committees, March 2021, https://www.gao.gov/assets/gao-21-248.pdf.

For a good paper describing that increased doses of naloxone are not needed to treat fentanyl overdoses, see J. Carpenter, B. P. Murray, S. Atti, T. P. Moran, A. Yancey, and B. Morgan, "Naloxone Dosing After Opioid

Overdose in the Era of Illicitly Manufactured Fentanyl," *Journal of Medical Toxicology* 16, no. 1 (January 2020): 41–48, https://doi.org/10.1007/s13181-019-00735-w.

This SWORD data shows no change in naloxone dosing by EMS over a four-year period: Connecticut Department of Public Health, "EMS Naloxone Administrations Per Patient 2020-2023," *CT EMS SWORD Statewide Opioid Reporting Directive Newsletter*, April 2023, 2–4, https://portal.ct.gov/-/media/Departments-and-Agencies/DPH/dph/ems/pdf/SWORD/SWORD-newsletters/2023/SWORDApril2023NL_FINALrev.pdf.

This controversial paper discusses the moral hazard of naloxone: Jennifer Doleac and Anita Mukherjee, "The Moral Hazard of Lifesaving Innovations: Naloxone Access, Opioid Abuse, and Crime," IZA DP No. 11489 (IZA Institute of Labor Economics, April 2019), https://docs.iza.org/dp11489.pdf.

These papers show the effectiveness of naloxone training: R. McDonald and J. Strang, "Are Take-Home Naloxone Programmes Effective? Systematic Review Utilizing Application of the Bradford Hill Criteria," *Addiction* 111, no. 7 (July 2016): 1177–87, https://doi.org/10.1111/add.13326; J. D. Jones, A. Campbell, V. E. Metz, S. D. Comer, "No Evidence of Compensatory Drug Use Risk Behavior among Heroin Users after Receiving Take-Home Naloxone," Addict Behav. 71 no. 00 (August 2017): 104–106, https://doi.org/ 10.1016/j.addbeh.2017.03.008.

For data from SUDORS, SWORD, and a research paper on previous overdoses and fatalities, see Centers for Disease Control and Prevention, "SUDORS Dashboard"; Connecticut Department of Public Health, *Statewide Opioid Reporting Directive (SWORD) 2021 Annual*

Report (Connecticut Department of Public Health, 2021), https://portal.ct.gov/-/media/departments-and-agencies/dph/dph/ems/pdf/sword/sword-newsletters/2021/second-sword-annual-report-slides.pdf; B. Suffoletto and A. Zeigler, "Risk and Protective Factors for Repeated Overdose After Opioid Overdose Survival," *Drug and Alcohol Dependence* 209 (April 1, 2020):107890, https://doi.org/10.1016/j.drugalcdep.2020.107890.

For SWORD data on patients requiring sedation post resuscitation see Connecticut Department of Public Health, "Patients Requiring EMS Sedation for Combativeness Post Naloxone," *CT EMS SWORD Statewide Opioid Reporting Directive Newsletter*, November 2022, https://portal.ct.gov/-/media/departments-and-agencies/dph/dph/ems/pdf/sword/sword-newsletters/2022/sworddec2022nl_final.pdf.

Chapter 4

This study details the low (but still real) risk of a second overdose immediately after resuscitation in those who reuse: Michael W. Willman, David B. Liss, Evan S. Schwarz, and Michael E. Mullins, "Do Heroin Overdose Patients Require Observation After Receiving Naloxone?" *Clinical Toxicology* 55, no. 2 (November 16, 2016): 81–87, https://doi.org/10.1080/15563650.2016.1253846.

This article describes the stigma many people who use drugs feel during visits to the ED: S. Mayer, V. Langheimer, S. Nolan, J. Boyd, W. Small, and R. McNeil, "Emergency Department Experiences of People Who Use Drugs Who Left or Were Discharged from Hospital Against Medical Advice," *PLoS One* 18, no. 2 (February 23, 2023): e0282215, https://doi.org/10.1371/journal.pone.0282215.

Recovery navigators in EDs are proving effective in assisting patients. See Eric G. Anderson, Evan Rusoja, Joshua Luftig, et al., "Effectiveness of Substance Use Navigation for Emergency Department Patients with Substance Use Disorders: An Implementation Study," *Annals of Emergency Medicine* 81, no. 3 (March 1, 2023): 297–308, https://doi.org/10.1016/j.annemergmed.2022.09.025.

Chapter 5

This fascinating paper explores the marketing behind oxycontin: A. Van Zee, "The Promotion and Marketing of OxyContin: Commercial Triumph, Public Health Tragedy," *American Journal of Public Health* 99, no. 2 (February 2009): 221–7, https://doi.org/10.2105/AJPH.2007.131714.

This paper contains a CDC graph illustrating prescription opioid overdoses: Centers for Disease Control and Prevention, "Vital Signs: Overdoses of Prescription Opioid Pain Relievers—United States, 1999–2008," *Morbidity and Mortality Weekly Report* 60, no. 43: 1487–92, https://www.cdc.gov/mmwr/preview/mmwrhtml/mm6043a4.htm.

This paper details the rise of heroin use: C. M. Jones, "Heroin Use and Heroin Use Risk Behaviors Among Nonmedical Users of Prescription Opioid Pain Relievers—United States, 2002–2004 and 2008–2010," *Drug and Alcohol Dependence* 132, no. 1–2 (2013): 95–100.

For DEA fentanyl facts detailing what is considered a lethal dose, see US Drug Enforcement Administration, "Facts About Fentanyl."

This article from PBS News discusses the Tylenol murders: Howard Markel, "How the Tylenol Murders of 1982 Changed the Way We Consume Medication," PBS News, September 29, 2014, https://www.pbs.org/newshour/health/tylenol-murders-1982.

The Connecticut Office of the Chief Medical Examiner releases detailed annual statistics on overdose deaths. See Connecticut Office of the Chief Medical Examiner, "Connecticut Accidental Drug Intoxication Deaths."

The 90 percent of heroin bags testing positive for fentanyl comes from the Greater Hartford Harm Reduction Coalition, who ran the project using fentanyl test strips. The CDC information is available here: M. F. Garnett and A. M. Miniño, "Drug Overdose Deaths in the United States, 2003–2023," 2024, https://doi.org/10.15620/cdc/170565.

Information on seized counterfeit pills comes from these sources: "Law Enforcement Seizures of Pills Containing Fentanyl Increased," National Institutes of Health, March 31, 2022, https://www.nih.gov/news-events/news-releases/law-enforcement-seizures-pills-containing-fentanyl-increased-dramatically-between-2018-2021; Drug Enforcement Administration, *National Drug Threat Assessment 2024* (DEA, 2024), https://www.dea.gov/sites/default/files/2024-07/2024%20NDTA-updated%207.5.2024.pdf; Drug Enforcement Administration, "One Pill Can Kill," DEA, n.d., https://www.dea.gov/onepill.

The following reports detail possible fentanyl-contaminated marijuana that many dispute: S. M. Nir, "Inside Fentanyl's Mounting Death Toll: 'This Is Poison,'" *New York Times*, November 22, 2021, https://www.nytimes.com/2021/11/20/nyregion/fentanyl-opioid-deaths.html; Sam Quinones, "Op-Ed: How Supply and Demand Have Driven the U.S. Drug Crisis Into the 'Synthetic Era,'" *Los Angeles Times*, October 31, 2021, https://www.latimes.com/opinion/story/2021-10-31/supply-demand-drug-crisis-synthetic.

These articles detail the Connecticut marijuana case and advisory: Seamus Mcavoy and Jesse Leavenworth, "Fentanyl-Laced Pot Confirmed in Connecticut for First Time, Caused OD in Plymouth," *Hartford Courant*,

November 19, 2021, https://www.courant.com/2021/11/18/fentanyl-laced-pot-confirmed-in-connecticut-for-first-time-caused-od-in-plymouth/; Samantha Simon, "Connecticut Falsely Linked Nearly 40 Overdoses to Fentanyl-Laced Marijuana, Report Finds," WSHU, February 3, 2022, https://www.wshu.org/connecticut-news/2022-02-02/connecticut-falsely-linked-nearly-40-overdoses-to-fentanyl-laced-marijuana-report-finds.

This article describes how fentanyl's burn point affects its potency when smoked with marijuana: Claire Zagorski, "The Pernicious Myth of Fentanyl-Laced Cannabis," Filter, July 20, 2021, https://filtermag.org/fentanyl-marijuana-myth/.

This paper explores the history of carfentanil in recent overdoses: H. Jalal and D. S. Burke, "Carfentanil and the Rise and Fall of Overdose Deaths in the United States," *Addiction* 116, no. 6 (June 2021): 1593–99, https://doi.org/10.1111/add.15260.

The SUDORS dashboard tracks various drugs, including carfentanil, nitazines, and xylazine: Centers for Disease Control and Prevention, "SUDORS Dashboard."

For articles on nitazines, see David Ovalle, "On the Streets, Opioids Sometimes More Potent Than Fentanyl: Nitazenes," *Washington Post*, December 22, 2023, https://www.washingtonpost.com/health/2023/12/10/nitazenes-opioid-stronger-than-fentanyl/; Centers for Disease Control and Prevention, "SUDORS Dashboard."

For articles on xylazine, see J. C. Reyes, J. L. Negrón, H. M. Colón, et al., "The Emerging of Xylazine as a New Drug of Abuse and Its Health Consequences Among Drug Users in Puerto Rico," *Journal of Urban Health* 89, no. 3 (June 2012): 519–26, https://doi.org/10.1007/s11524-011-9662-6; Laura Strickler, "This State Is Counting the Human Casualties from a Drug Meant for Animals," NBC News, December 10, 2023, https://news.yahoo.com/news/state-counting-human-casualties-drug-140000110.html?fr=sycsrp_catchall; S. Choi, M. R. Irwin, and E. A. Kiyatkin, "Xylazine Effects on Opioid-Induced Brain Hypoxia," *Psychopharmacology* 240 (2023), 1561–71, https://doi.org/10.1007/s00213-023-06390-y; Drug Enforcement Administration, "The Growing Threat of Xylazine and Its Mixture with Illicit Drugs," DEA, December 21, 2022, https://www.dea.gov/documents/2022/2022-12/2022-12-21/growing-threat-xylazine-and-its-mixture-illicit-drugs.

For a key study that suggests that adding xylazine to a street mix might actually lead to less-severe overdoses, see J. S. Love, M. Levine, K. Aldy, et al., "Opioid Overdoses Involving Xylazine in Emergency Department Patients: A Multicenter Study," *Clinical Toxicology* 61, no. 3 (March 2023): 173–80, https://doi.org/10.1080/15563650.2022.2159427.

For Connecticut OCME stats on xylazine in deaths, see Connecticut Office of the Chief Medical Examiner, "Connecticut Accidental Drug Intoxication Deaths."

Example of xylazine hysteria is in the senator's press release: "Schumer: Xylazine, a Deadly Skin-Rotting Zombie Drug, Often Mixed w Fentanyl, Is on the Doorstep of Cortland & Onondaga Counties, Already Fueling a Horrific Wave of Overdoses & Deaths Across Central NY; Senator Will Launch Three-Pronged Plan to Cut Off Supply, Aid Local Law Enforcement, & Bolster Addiction Services to Combat Overdose Epidemic," Chuck Schumer's official website, March 10, 2023, https://www.schumer.senate.gov/newsroom/press-releases/schumer-xylazine-a-deadly-skin-rotting-zombie-drug-often-mixed-w-fentanyl-is-on-the-doorstep-of-cortland-and-onondaga-counties-already-fueling-a-horrific-wave-of-overdoses_deaths-across-central-ny-senator-will-launch-three-pronged-plan-to-cut-off-supply-aid-local-law-enforcement--bolster-addiction-services-to-combat-overdose-epidemic.

Hysteria over fentanyl has often derived from reports of police exposure. See, for example, B. Del Pozo, J. D. Rich, and J. J. Carroll, "Reports of Accidental Fentanyl Overdose Among Police in the Field: Toward Correcting a Harmful Culture-Bound Syndrome," *International Journal of Drug Policy* 100 (February 2022):103520, https://doi.org/10.1016/j.drugpo.2021.103520.

For information on how fentanyl works transdermally with special skin patches, see Mayo Clinic, "Fentanyl (Transdermal Route)," updated October 1, 2024, https://www.mayoclinic.org/drugs-supplements/fentanyl-transdermal-route/proper-use/drg-20068152.

For more material on the false narrative that just touching fentanyl can cause overdose, see US Department of Justice, "Roll Call Video Warns About Dangers of Fentanyl Exposure," US Department of Justice, May 27, 2022, https://www.justice.gov/opa/video/roll-call-video-warns-about-dangers-fentanyl-exposure; M. J. Moss, B. J. Warrick, L. S. Nelson, et al., "ACMT and AACT Position Statement: Preventing Occupational Fentanyl and Fentanyl Analog Exposure to Emergency Responders," *Journal of Medical Toxicology* 13, no. 4 (2017): 347–51, https://doi.org/10.1007/s13181-017-0628-2; Bureau of Justice Assistance, "Fentanyl: The Real Deal," Bureau of Justice Assistance, November 24, 2019, https://bja.ojp.gov/fentanyl-real-deal.

For examples of overblown news stories, see Quinn Owen, "DEA Seized Enough Fentanyl to Kill Every American in 2022," ABC News, December 21, 2022, https://abcnews.go.com/Politics/dea-seized-fentanyl-kill-american-2022/story?id=95625574; Drug Enforcement Administration, "DEA Warns of Brightly-Colored Fentanyl Used to Target Young Americans," DEA, August 30, 2022, https://www.dea.gov/press-releases/2022/08/30/dea-warns-brightly-colored-fentanyl-used-target-young-americans.

For the story of the toddler who died after getting into a drug stash, see M. Cramer, "2 Charged with Murder in Day Care Death of 1-Year-Old," *New York Times*, September 17, 2023. https://www.nytimes.com/2023/09/17/nyregion/opioid-bronx-daycare-fentanyl-murder-charge.html.

For SWORD data on youth overdoses, see Connecticut Department of Public Health and Office of Emergency Medical Services, "Annual SWORD Data Review," *CT EMS SWORD Statewide Opioid Reporting Directive Newsletter*, February 2023, https://portal.ct.gov/-/media/departments-and-agencies/dph/dph/ems/pdf/sword/sword-newsletters/2023/swordfeb2023nl_finalrev.pdf.

For articles promoting the fourth wave of the opioid epidemic theory, see, for example, Richard A. Rawson, Tyler G. Erath, and H. Westley Clark, "The Fourth Wave of the Overdose Crisis: Examining the Prominent Role of Psychomotor Stimulants with and Without Fentanyl," *Preventive Medicine* 176 (November 1, 2023): 107625, https://doi.org/10.1016/j.ypmed.2023.107625; J. Friedman and C. L. Shover, "Charting the Fourth Wave: Geographic, Temporal, Race/Ethnicity and Demographic Trends in Polysubstance Fentanyl Overdose Deaths in the United States, 2010–2021," *Addiction* 118, no. 12 (2023): 2477–85, https://doi.org/10.1111/add.16318.

For Connecticut OCME data on the rise of cocaine presence in fatal opioid cases, see Connecticut Office of the Chief Medical Examiner, "Connecticut Accidental Drug Intoxication Deaths."

Chapter 6

For more on the origins of opium, see "Origins and History of Opium," Herb Museum, 1994. http://www.herbmuseum.ca/content/origins-and-history-opium.

Tennyson's poem can be found here: Alfred Lord Tennyson, "The Lotos-Eaters," Poetry Foundation, https://www.poetryfoundation.org/poems/45364/the-lotos-eaters.

Here is a fascinating conversation between a leading substance use scholar and a harm reduction activist: "Dr. Gabor Maté and Former Patient Guy Felicella Talk Trauma, Addiction, & Recovery," interview by Guy Felicella, posted December 13, 2023, by ethno., YouTube, https://www.youtube.com/watch?v=B-UojfNzorE.

Some of the information I share about Austin Eubanks came from attending one of his talks. Here is an article about his death and life: Weisfeldt, S., and Vera, A., "Columbine shooting survivor Austin Eubanks died of a heroin overdose," *CNN*, June 14, 2019, https://www.cnn.com/2019/06/13/us/columbine-survivor-austin-eubanks-heroin-overdose-trnd/index.html.

For an explanation of substance use disorder from the American Psychiatric Association, see American Psychiatric Association, "What Is a Substance Use Disorder?" American Psychiatric Association, n.d., https://www.psychiatry.org/patients-families/addiction/what-is-addiction.

For the definition of addiction from the American Society of Addiction Medicine, see American Society of Addiction Medicine, "Public Policy Statement: Definition of Addiction," American Society of Addiction Medicine, July 15, 2011, https://www.asam.org/docs/default-source/quality-science/asam%27s-2019-definition-of-addiction-(1).pdf?sfvrsn=b8b64fc2_2.

A great explanation of how addiction works can be found in this book: Substance Abuse and Mental Health Services Administration, Office of the Surgeon General, *Facing Addiction in America: The Surgeon*

General's Report on Alcohol, Drugs, and Health (US Department of Health and Human Services, 2016), https://www.ncbi.nlm.nih.gov/books/NBK424857/.

Chapter 7

For statistics from the National Institute on Drug Abuse on the number of people with substance use disorder who are receiving treatment, see "Only 1 in 5 U.S. Adults with Opioid Use Disorder Received Medications to Treat It in 2021," National Institute on Drug Abuse, August 7, 2023, https://nida.nih.gov/news-events/news-releases/2023/08/only-1-in-5-us-adults-with-opioid-use-disorder-received-medications-to-treat-it-in-2021.

Relapse is a part of recovery for many chronic diseases, including substance use disorder. See National Institute on Drug Abuse, "Treatment and Recovery," National Institute on Drug Abuse, July 6, 2020, https://nida.nih.gov/publications/drugs-brains-behavior-science-addiction/treatment-recovery.

Information on detoxification came from the SAMSA: Substance Abuse and Mental Health Services Administration, "Overview, Essential Concepts, and Definitions in Detoxification," chap. 1 in *Detoxification and Substance Abuse Treatment* (Substance Abuse and Mental Health Services Administration, 2006), https://www.ncbi.nlm.nih.gov/books/NBK64119/.

The cost of drug rehab information came from the National Center for Drug Abuse Statistics: "Average Cost of Drug Rehab," NCDAS, March 25, 2024, https://drugabusestatistics.org/cost-of-rehab/.

For an article about low rates of buprenorphine misuse, see Beth Han, Christopher M. Jones, Emily B. Einstein, and Wilson M. Compton,

"Trends in and Characteristics of Buprenorphine Misuse Among Adults in the US," *JAMA Network Open* 4, no. 10 (October 15, 2021): e2129409, https://doi.org/10.1001/jamanetworkopen.2021.29409.

For a great paper on the effectiveness of opioid agonists on the death rate in Baltimore, see R. P. Schwartz, J. Gryczynski, K. E. O'Grady, et al., "Opioid Agonist Treatments and Heroin Overdose Deaths in Baltimore, Maryland, 1995–2009," *American Journal of Public Health* 103, no. 5 (May 2013): 917–22, https://doi.org/10.2105/AJPH.2012.301049.

For sources on methadone and Suboxone information and barriers to care, see Substance Abuse and Mental Health Services Administration, "Substance Use Disorder Treatment Options," SAMHSA, updated April 11, 2024, https://www.samhsa.gov/substance-use/treatment/options; World Health Organization, "WHO Model Lists of Essential Medicines," WHO.int, n.d., https://www.who.int/groups/expert-committee-on-selection-and-use-of-essential-medicines/essential-medicines-lists; Christopher M. Jones, Beth Han, Grant T. Baldwin, Emily B. Einstein, and Wilson M. Compton, "Use of Medication for Opioid Use Disorder Among Adults with Past-Year Opioid Use Disorder in the US, 2021," *JAMA Network Open* 6, no. 8 (August 7, 2023): e2327488, https://doi.org/10.1001/jamanetworkopen.2023.27488; E. Hutchinson, M. Catlin, C. H. Andrilla, L. M. Baldwin, and R. A. Rosenblatt, "Barriers to Primary Care Physicians Prescribing Buprenorphine," *Annals of Family Medicine* 12, no. 2 (March–April 2014): 128–33, https://doi.org/10.1370/afm.1595; Health and Human Services Department, "Medications for the Treatment of Opioid Use Disorder," Federal Register, February 2, 2024, https://www.federalregister.gov/documents/2024/02/02/2024-01693/medications-for-the-treatment-of-opioid-use-disorder; W. C. Goedel, A. Shapiro, M. Cerdá, J. W. Tsai, S. E. Hadland, and B. D. L. Marshall, "Association of Racial/Ethnic Segregation with Treatment Capacity for Opioid Use Disorder in Counties in the United States," *JAMA Network Open* 3, no. 4 (2020): e203711, https://doi.org/10.1001/jamanetworkopen.2020.3711; Clare Stroud, Sheena M. Posey Norris, and Lisa Bain, "The History of Methadone and Barriers to Access for Different Populations," chap. 3 in *Methadone Treatment for Opioid Use Disorder* (National Academies Press, July 15, 2022), https://www.ncbi.nlm.nih.gov/books/NBK585210/.

For natrexone's effect on patients craving opioids, see B. A. G. Dijkstra, C. A. J. De Jong, S. M. Bluschke, et al., "Does Naltrexone Affect Craving in Abstinent Opioid-Dependent Patients?" *Addiction Biology* 12, no. 2 (May 14, 2007): 176–82, https://doi.org/10.1111/j.1369-1600.2007.00067.x

Treatment options can be further explored here: Treatment Atlas, "National Principles of Care," Shatterproof, https://treatmentatlas.org/national-principles-care.

For more on the high cost of opioid use disorder and the small amount we spend on treatment, see Centers for Disease Control and Prevention, "Cost of Injury & Violence," Centers for Disease Control and Prevention, September 19, 2023, https://www.cdc.gov/injury-violence-prevention/economics/?CDC_AAref_Val=https://www.cdc.gov/injury/features/health-econ-cost-of-injury/index.html.

Chapter 8

I am not a big X fan, but I always read this gentleman's posts. He is an ardent advocate for harm reduction and human dignity. Guy Felicella (guyfelicellaCA@guyfelicella), https://x.com/guyfelicella.

Van Asher is a former EMT and harm reductionist who is also one of my heroes. His YouTube channel is a great explanation of harm reduction: Van Asher, "Harm Reduction and Abstinence Based Treatment,

'Bridging the Gap,'" posted February 22, 2022, by Van Asher, Harm Reduction Page, YouTube, https://www.youtube.com/watch?v=gunPqQuZz4Y.

Money spent on prevention pays dividends financially and in human health. See T. Q. Nguyen, B. W. Weir, D. C. Des Jarlais, S. D. Pinkerton, and D. R. Holtgrave, "Syringe Exchange in the United States: A National Level Economic Evaluation of Hypothetical Increases in Investment," *AIDS and Behavior* 18, no. 11 (November 2014): 2144–55, https://doi.org/10.1007/s10461-014-0789-9; "Safety and effectiveness of syringe services programs," Syringe Services Programs (SSPs), February 8, 2024, https://www.cdc.gov/syringe-services-programs/php/safety-effectiveness.html?CDC_AAref_Val=https://www.cdc.gov/ssp/syringe-services-programs-summary.html.

Overdose prevention has proven to save lives. See B. D. Marshall, M. J. Milloy, E. Wood, J. S. Montaner, and T. Kerr, "Reduction in Overdose Mortality After the Opening of North America's First Medically Supervised Safer Injecting Facility: A Retrospective Population-Based Study," *Lancet* 377, no. 9775 (April 2011):1429–37, https://doi.org/10.1016/S0140-6736(10)62353-7; H. Hagan, J. P. McGough, H. Thiede, S. Hopkins, J. Duchin, and E. R. Alexander, "Reduced Injection Frequency and Increased Entry and Retention in Drug Treatment Associated with Needle-Exchange Participation in Seattle Drug Injectors," *Journal of Substance Abuse Treatment* 19, no. 3 (October 2000): 247–52, https://doi.org/10.1016/s0740-5472(00)00104-5; A. Irwin, E. Jozaghi, B. W. Weir, S. Allen, A. Lindsay, S. Sherman, "Mitigating the Heroin Crisis in Baltimore, MD, USA: A Cost-Benefit Analysis of a Hypothetical Supervised Injection Facility," *Harm Reduction Journal* 14, 29 (2017), https://doi.org/10.1186/s12954-017-0153-2.

Chapter 9

Stigma against people who use drugs is a powerful negative force on society and people's lives. See Centers for Disease Control and Prevention, "SUDORS Dashboard"; R. Room, "Stigma, Social Inequality and Alcohol and Drug Use," *Drug and Alcohol Review*, 24 (2005): 143–55, https://doi.org/10.1080/09595230500102434.

The World Health Organization study of stigma is cited here: M. Kulesza, S. Ramsey, R. Brown, M. Larimer, "Stigma among Individuals with Substance Use Disorders: Does It Predict Substance Use, and Does It Diminish with Treatment?" *Journal of Addictive Behaviors, Therapy and Rehabilitation* 3 (January 15, 2014): 1000115, http://dx.doi.org/10.4172/2324-9005.1000115.

Zombie language generates clicks and hate. See J. Raasch, "'Zombie Apocalypse': San Francisco on Track to Crush Overdose Death Record as Addicts Die in Streets," Fox News, September 25, 2023, https://www.foxnews.com/us/zombie-apocalypse-san-francisco-track-crush-overdose-death-record-addicts-die-streets; "Skin Rotting 'Zombie Drug' Causes Havoc Across the US Cities," posted February 25, 2023, by the Free Press Journal, YouTube, https://youtu.be/ZGuKuzr_070.

For a fascinating study on stigma, see Nora D. Volkow, "Stigma and the Toll of Addiction," *New England Journal of Medicine* 382, no. 14 (April 2, 2020): 1289–90, https://doi.org/10.1056/nejmp1917360.

The Associated Press has made efforts to improve journalistic coverage of the substance use crisis by stopping the use of stigmatizing language. See L. G. Bessette, S. C. Hauc, H. Danckers, A. Atayde, and R. Saitz, "The Associated Press Stylebook Changes and the Use of Addiction-Related

Stigmatizing Terms in News Media," *Substance Abuse* 43, no. 1 (2022): 127–30, https://doi.org/10.1080/08897077.2020.1748167.

For headlines from my local paper, see Alison Cross, "'Zombie Drug' Hits Connecticut with Devastating Impact. Here's Why It's Gaining Traction," *Hartford Courant*, September 5, 2023, https://www.courant.com/2023/09/04/modern-day-leprosy-xylazine-hits-connecticut-with-devastating-impact.

This fascinating article explores the subject of much debate in the harm reduction community: Keith Humphreys and Jonathan Caulkins, "Destigmatizing Drug Use Has Been a Profound Mistake," *The Atlantic*, December 13, 2023, https://www.theatlantic.com/ideas/archive/2023/12/destigmatizing-drug-use-mistake-opioid-crisis/676292.

Chapter 10

For Supreme Court Justice William O. Douglas's landmark ruling in Robinson v. California, see "Robinson V. California, 370 U.S. 660 (1962)," Justia Law, n.d., https://supreme.justia.com/cases/federal/us/370/660/.

This great article from the *New York Times* shows the insanity of how many treat the opioid crisis: Eli Salslow, "He Tried to Save a Friend: They Charged Him with Murder," *New York Times*, September 28, 2023, https://www.nytimes.com/2023/06/25/us/fentanyl-murder-charge.html.

Addiction is not as easy as a simple choice. Science is key to understanding addiction. See J. Suckling and L. J. Nestor, "The Neurobiology of Addiction: The Perspective from Magnetic Resonance Imaging Present and

Future," *Addiction* 112, no. 2 (February 2017): 360–69, https://doi.org/10.1111/add.13474.

This comprehensive book discusses the role of the Sackler family and pharma in creating the opioid crisis: P. Radden Keefe, *Empire of Pain: The Secret History of the Sackler Dynasty* (Picador, 2021).

Again, dollars spent on prevention could save far more down the road. When will we learn? See Centers for Disease Control and Prevention, "Cost of Injury & Violence," Centers for Disease Control and Prevention, September 19, 2023, https://www.cdc.gov/injury-violence-prevention/economics/?CDC_AAref_Val=https://www.cdc.gov/injury/features/health-econ-cost-of-injury/index.html; Frank Wilczek and *Quanta Magazine*, "Einstein's Parable of Quantum Insanity," *Scientific American*, February 20, 2024, https://www.scientificamerican.com/article/einstein-s-parable-of-quantum-insanity/.

What if politicians looked out for the good of the country instead of trying to target their opponents? What great pain might have been avoided? See, for example, D. Baum, "Legalize it All," *Harpers*, https://harpers.org/archive/2016/04/legalize-it-all/; "Cracks in the System: 20 Years of the Unjust Federal Crack Cocaine Law," American Civil Liberties Union, October 25, 2006, https://www.aclu.org/documents/cracks-system-20-years-unjust-federal-crack-cocaine-law; National Institutes of Health, "Criminal Justice DrugFacts," National Institute on Drug Abuse, March 23, 2023, https://nida.nih.gov/publications/drugfacts/criminal-justice.

A person serves their time and then is released into an unforgiving world. Those released from prison are at terrible risk for overdose death. See, for example, I. A. Binswanger, M. F. Stern, R. A. Deyo RA, et al., "Release from Prison—A High Risk of Death for Former Inmates," *New*

England Journal of Medicine 356, no. 2 (January 2007): 157–65, https://doi.org/10.1056/NEJMsa064115. Erratum in: *New England Journal of Medicine* 356, no. 5 (February 2007): 536.

Too often we might base policy on what sounds good on the political stump, not on what works. For more information on this, see M. Peterson, J. Rich, A. Macmadu, et al., "One Guy Goes to Jail, Two People Are Ready to Take His Spot": Perspectives on Drug-Induced Homicide Laws Among Incarcerated Individuals," *International Journal of Drug Policy* 70 (August 2019): 47–53, https://doi.org/10.1016/j.drugpo.2019.05.001; Christopher J. Mumola and Jennifer C. Karberg, *Drug Use and Dependence, State and Federal Prisoners, 2004* (Bureau of Justice Statistics, 2006, revised January 19, 2007), https://bjs.ojp.gov/content/pub/pdf/dudsfp04.pdf; B. Ray, S. J. Korzeniewski, G. Mohler, et al., "Spatiotemporal Analysis Exploring the Effect of Law Enforcement Drug Market Disruptions on Overdose, Indianapolis, Indiana, 2020–2021," *American Journal of Public Health* 113, no. 7 (July 1, 2023): 750–58, https://doi.org/10.2105/ajph.2023.307291; Bryce Pardo and Peter Reuter, "Enforcement Strategies for Fentanyl and Other Synthetic Opioids," Brookings Institution, June 22, 2020, https://www.brookings.edu/articles/enforcement-strategies-for-fentanyl-and-other-synthetic-opioids/.

Who would believe a cartel boss? See Jose de Cordoba, "Mexican Sinaloa Cartel's Message to Members: Stop Making Fentanyl or Die," *Wall Street Journal*, October 16, 2023, https://www.wsj.com/world/americas/mexican-sinaloa-cartels-message-to-members-stop-making-fentanyl-or-die-b96d3e09; Drug Enforcement Administration, *National Drug Threat Assessment 2024 National Drug Threat Assessment 2024* (DEA, February 2024), https://www.dea.gov/sites/default/files/2024-07/2024%20NDTA-updated%207.5.2024.pdf.

Efforts to target precursor chemicals are not guaranteed to work long term but are worth trying. See White House, "Memorandum on Prioritizing the Strategic Disruption of the Supply Chain for Illicit Fentanyl and Synthetic Opioids Through a Coordinated, Whole-of-Government, Information-Driven Effort," July 21, 2024, https://bidenwhitehouse.archives.gov/briefing-room/presidential-actions/2024/07/31/memorandum-on-prioritizing-the-strategic-disruption-of-the-supply-chain-for-illicit-fentanyl-and-synthetic-opioids-through-a-coordinated-whole-of-government-information-driven-effort/; B. Mann, "Critics Wary as China Promises Tighter Fentanyl Control," NPR, August 30, 2024, https://www.npr.org/2024/08/29/nx-s1-5089978/fentanyl-china-precursors.

There have been recent reports of the street supply containing less fentanyl. Hopefully, this is not just a blip but lasting progress. See, for example, B. Mann, "The Street Supply of Fentanyl Is Dropping. This Shift Could Save Thousands," NPR, October 1, 2024, https://www.npr.org/2024/10/01/nx-s1-5132067/the-street-supply-of-fentanyl-is-dropping-this-shift-could-save-thousands.

It's time to look at other strategies to save lives. See, for example, A. Ivsins, J. Boyd, L. Beletsky, and R. McNeil, "Tackling the Overdose Crisis: The Role of Safe Supply," *International Journal of Drug Policy* 80 (June 2020): 102769, https://doi.org/10.1016/j.drugpo.2020.102769; Holly Hedegaard, Arialdi M. Miniño, and Margaret Warner, "Drug Overdose Deaths in the United States, 2001–2021," Centers for Disease Control and Prevention, December 22, 2022, https://doi.org/10.15620/cdc:122556.

Decriminalization should be considered nationwide. See Drug Policy Alliance, "Approaches to Decriminalizing Drug Use & Possession,"

United Nations Office on Drugs and Crime, February 2015, https://www.unodc.org/documents/ungass2016/Contributions/Civil/DrugPolicyAlliance/DPA_Fact_Sheet_Approaches_to_Decriminalization_Feb2015_1.pdf; United Nations Economic and Social Council, Commission on Narcotic Drugs, https://www.unodc.org/documents/commissions/CND/CND_Sessions/CND_60/NGO_Papers/ECN72017_NGO5_V1701416.pdf; Transform Drug Policy Foundation, "Drug Decriminalization in Portugal: Setting the Record Straight," Transform Drug Policy Foundation, May 13, 2021, https://transformdrugs.org/blog/drug-decriminalisation-in-portugal-setting-the-record-straight; Morgan Godvin, "Don't Blame Drug Decriminalization for What the Housing Crisis Has Caused," Truthout, August 12, 2023, https://truthout.org/articles/dont-blame-drug-decriminalization-for-what-the-housing-crisis-has-caused/.

Solving homelessness and other root causes that may drive people to substance use need to be addressed. See Nicholas Kristof, "Here's How Houston Is Fighting Homelessness—and Winning," *New York Times*, November 22, 2023, https://www.nytimes.com/2023/11/22/opinion/homeless-houston-dallas.html.

Just say no and drug lectures don't work. Nor does mandating someone to treatment. See, for example, D. Werb, A. Kamarulzaman, M. C. Meacham, et al., "The Effectiveness of Compulsory Drug Treatment: A Systematic Review," *International Journal of Drug Policy* 28 (February 2016): 1–9, https://doi.org/10.1016/j.drugpo.2015.12.005.

For a provocative article on legalization, see D. Baum, "Legalize It All," *Harper's*, April 2016, https://archive.harpers.org/2016/04/pdf/HarpersMagazine-2016-04-0085915.pdf.

Politics and appeals to fear rather than true solutions take the day at election time. See, for example, M. Smith, "What Do These Political Ads Have in Common? The Opioid Crisis," *New York Times*, June 7, 2018, https://www.nytimes.com/2018/06/07/us/opioid-ads-democrats-republicans.html.

Epilogue

Overdoses are declining in Connecticut and nationwide. See F. B. Ahmad, J. A. Cisewski, L. M. Rossen, and P. Sutton, "Provisional Drug Overdose Death Counts," National Center for Health Statistics, updated January 15, 2025, https://www.cdc.gov/nchs/nvss/vsrr/drug-overdose-data.htm.

To read the Hippocratic oath, see "Hippocratic Oath," Wikipedia, last modified November 23, 2024, https://en.wikipedia.org/wiki/Hippocratic_Oath.

Action Plan

Fentanyl represented 88 percent of all opioid deaths in 2021. See Centers for Disease Control "U.S. overdose deaths in 2021 increased half as much as in 2020 - but are still up 15%." May 11, 2022. https://www.cdc.gov/nchs/pressroom/nchs_press_releases/2022/202205.htm.

There is a great *New York Times* article that discusses the debate over the terms *overdose* versus *poisoning*: J. Hoffman, "Overdose or Poisoning? A New Debate over What to Call a Drug Death," *New York Times*, March 11, 2024, https://www.nytimes.com/2024/03/11/health/overdose-poison-fentanyl.html.

CDC data shows a hopeful decline in deaths: B. Mann, "NPR Exclusive: U.S. Overdose Deaths Plummet, Saving Thousands of Lives," NPR, September 18, 2024, https://www.npr.org/2024/09/18/nx-s1-5107417/overdose-fatal-fentanyl-death-opioid; Ahmad et al., "Provisional Drug Overdose Death Counts."

Glossary

This is an excellent review of the genetics behind substance use disorder: J. D. Deak and E. C. Johnson, "Genetics of Substance Use Disorders: A Review," *Psychological Medicine* 51 no. 13 (2021): 2189–2200. https://doi.org/10.1017/s0033291721000969.

For an interesting article on the effects of prohibition, see Sarah Beller, "Infographic: The 'Iron Law of Prohibition,'" *Filter*, October 3, 2018, https://filtermag.org/infographic-the-iron-law-of-prohibition/.

Black deaths are rising. We need to keep addressing this with every bit of urgency as white deaths. See Mbabazi Kariisa et al., "*Vital Signs*: Drug Overdose Deaths, by Selected Sociodemographic and Social Determinants of Health Characteristics—25 States and the District of Columbia, 2019–2020," *Morbidity and Mortality Weekly Report* 71, no. 29 (July 22, 2022): 940–47, https://doi.org/10.15585/mmwr.mm7129e2.

Insite, the first safe injection site in Canada, has been a great success in preventing overdose death. See Vancouver Coastal Health, "Canada's First Supervised Consumption Site Celebrates 20 Years of Saving Lives," September 14, 2023, https://www.vch.ca/en/news/canadas-first-supervised-consumption-site-celebrates-20-years-saving-lives.

A federal court ruled against Philadelphia Safehouse efforts to establish a safe injection site. See N. Feldman, "In Philadelphia, Judges Rule against

Opening 'Supervised' Site to Inject Opioids," *NPR*, 2021, https://www.npr.org/sections/health-shots/2021/01/14/956428659/in-philadelphia-judges-rule-against-opening-a-medical-site-to-safely-inject-hero.

For more on substance use and mental disorders, see "Substance Use and Co-Occurring Mental Disorders," National Institute of Mental Health, March 2024, https://www.nimh.nih.gov/health/topics/substance-use-and-mental-health.

ABOUT THE AUTHOR

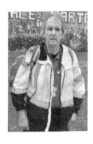

Peter Canning has been a paramedic in Hartford, Connecticut, since January 1995. His first book, *Paramedic: On the Front Lines of Medicine* (1997), details his journey from speechwriter for the governor of Connecticut to caregiver on the city streets. *Rescue 471: A Paramedic's Stories* (2000) is the sequel. *Killing Season: A Paramedic's Dispatches from the Front Lines of the Opioid Epidemic* was published by Johns Hopkins University Press and selected by Amazon as one of the ten best nonfiction books of April 2021.

Canning is also the author of two EMS novels, *Mortal Men* (2012) and *Diamond in the Rough* (2016), and the short story collection *Promised Land* (1994). Since 2006, he has written the influential EMS blog Streetwatch: Notes of a Paramedic (www.medicscribe.com). Writing as "Medicscribe," he posts regularly about the opioid epidemic and other topics from an EMS perspective.

A graduate of the Iowa Writers' Workshop, Canning attended Phillips Exeter Academy and the University of Virginia. He has worked many jobs in his life: tennis instructor, aide to a United States senator, taxi driver, meat-packer, line cook, telephone solicitor, book and movie reviewer, factory worker, health department administrator, speechwriter, and political campaign director before finding his place in life as a paramedic. In addition to being a field paramedic, he is the EMS coordinator at UConn John Dempsey Hospital in Farmington, Connecticut.

Canning lives in West Hartford with his wife, Chevaughn, and their three children.

Website: www.petercanning.org
Blog: www.medicscribe.com
Instagram: Peter Canning (@medicscribe)
X: Peter Canning (@medicscribe)

ILLUSTRATION CREDITS

vi Connecticut Harm Reduction Alliance
xi Photo by the author
3 Author figure
18 Today I Matter, Inc.
33 Photo by the author
46 Photo by the author
71 Photo by the author
88 DEA
97 Photo by the author
99 DEA
115 Photo by the author
126 Photo by the author
140 Connecticut Harm Reduction Alliance
151 Photo by the author
164 Today I Matter, Inc.
181 Connecticut Harm Reduction Alliance
192 Today I Matter, Inc.
194 Connecticut Harm Reduction Alliance
195 Connecticut Harm Reduction Alliance
249 Photo by Jerry Sneed

INDEX

Illustrations are indicated by page numbers in italics.

abstinence, 28–29, 163, 183, 201
access to opioids, as risk factor, 21–22
ACEs. *See* adverse childhood experiences (ACEs)
addict, defined, 201. *See also* junkie
addiction: defined, 118, 201; as disease, 9–10, 120–21, 125–27, 165; journeys into, 7, 9; prevalence of, 11; relapse in, 125, 127; risk factors, 20–26; science of, 118–21; stigma and, 150. *See also* treatment, of addiction
admission, to hospital, 79–80
adulteration, of opioids, 8, 88–93
adverse childhood experiences (ACEs), as risk factor, 23
age, as risk factor, 25–26
age at first use, as risk factor, 22–23
agitation, 75
agonal breathing, 37
alcohol, 26, 45, 57, 116, 175
alone, as risk factor, 29–30
assessment, post-resuscitation, 74–76

atomizer, for naloxone, 50–52
auto-injector, 52

Baltimore, Maryland, 146–47
behavioral therapy, 130
benzodiazepines, 26, 45, 57, 201
Biden, Joe, 143
bioavailability, 39, 202
Blumenthal, Richard, 176
boofing, 38–39
brain injury, from oxygen deprivation, 80
breathing, 32–34, 36–37, 40–41, 54, 79–80
Bruce, Lenny, 119
buprenorphine, 19, 76, 78–79, 131–33, 202. *See also* medication-assisted treatment (MAT)

carbon dioxide, 33–34
cardiac arrest, 32–33, 55, 73–74
carfentanil, 102–3, 170, 202
cartels, 170–71
Caulkins, Jonathan, 157–58
central nervous system, 32
childhood trauma, 10, 23
children: myths about fentanyl and, 110–11; overdose in, 25

choking, 36, 41
CMO. *See* comfort measures only (CMO)
coach, recovery, 210
cocaine, 22, 24, 91, 100–101, 111–12, 167–68, 203
Columbine High School shooting, 117–18
comfort measures only (CMO), 80
comorbidities, 203
costs: of opioid epidemic, 166; of treatment programs, 119; of War on Drugs, 213
counterfeit prescription drugs, 21–22, 98–99, *99*
courts, drug, 205
COVID pandemic, 133, 203–4
Cowan, Richard, 206
CPR (cardiopulmonary resuscitation), 2, 54–55, 74
crack cocaine, 167–68
crack house statute, 142–43
cutting, of opioids, 8, 88–93
cyanosis, 34, 36–37

death rattle, 37
deaths, overdose: abstinence and, 28–29; in children, 25; fentanyl in, 8; harm reduction and, 146; increase in, *3*, 171–72; injection and, 27–28; numbers, 96
decriminalization, 172–75, 204
dependence, 65, 204. *See also* addiction

detoxification, 127–29, 205
discrimination, stigma and, 155
disposition, from hospital, 79
dopamine, 119–20
Douglas, William O., 163
drug courts, 205

Ehrlichman, John, 166–67
EMS. *See* first responders
epinephrine, 73
Eubanks, Austin, 117–18

Felicella, Guy, 117, 144
fentanyl: as adulterant in heroin, 8, 88–91; adulteration of, 92–93; defined, 205; illicit sources of, 89–90; length of high from, 91; lethal dose of, *88*; lipophilicity of, 91–92; myths about, 107–11; in opioid crisis, 87–112; in palliative care, 89; potency of, 1, 8; Sinaloa cartel and, 170–71; test strips, 95–96, *97*; in 2021 overdose deaths, 8; unsafe supply of, 93; withdrawal, 91–92
first responders, 72–76, 140–41
fourth wave, of opioid epidemic, 111–12

gag reflex, 36
gender, as risk factor, 25
genetics, as risk factor, 24–25
Good Samaritan laws, 62–63

harm reduction: cost-benefit analysis with, 146–47; crack house statute and, 142–43; deaths and, 146; defined, 205–6; examples in medicine, 139; examples in opioid addiction, 61; naloxone and, 79; outreach, 140; typical services in, 144–45
heroin: adulteration of, 92–93; defined, 206; fentanyl as adulterant in, 8, 88–91; fentanyl as stronger than, 1; history of, 115–16; length of high from, 91; in opioid crisis, 87–88; OxyContin and, 87–88
history of substance use, as risk factor, 22
HIV, 79, 132, 146, 173
homelessness, 173–74
Homer, 114
hospital, 76–79
housing assistance, 19–20
Humphreys, Keith, 157–58
hydromorphone, 171
hypoxia, 34, 80

impulsivity, 24
infants, 25
injection: of naloxone, 52–53; of opioids, 27–28, 39
In the Realm of Hungry Ghost: Close Encounters with Addiction (Maté), 116–17
iron law of prohibition, 206

Jenkins, Mark, 141–42, 145–46, *181*, 184
junkie, 143, 150, 153–55, 157, 176, 206. *See also* stigma

Killing Season: A Paramedic's Dispatches from the Front Lines of the Opioid Epidemic (Canning), 8–9, 183
Kloxxado. *See* naloxone

legalization, 175–77, 207
lipophilicity, 91–92
"Lotos-Eaters, The" (Tennyson), 114

marijuana, 22, 101–2, 143
Maslow's hierarchy of needs, 120
MAT. *See* medication-assisted treatment (MAT)
Maté, Gabor, 116–17
media, stigma and, 157
medication-assisted treatment (MAT), 130–32, 147, 207. *See also* buprenorphine; hydromorphone; methadone
Mendell, Gary, 135–36
mental health, as risk factor, 23–24
methadone, 19, 125–26, 131, 133–34, 207. *See also* medication-assisted treatment (MAT)
methamphetamine, 27, 45, 91, 111, 117, 207
method of action, 32–34
miosis, 35

morphine, 39, 89, 115–16, 207–8
Murray, Stephen, 101

nalmefene, 50
naloxone, 1, 4–5, 9; administration of, 47–53; defined, 208; drugs resistant to, 45, 57; expiration of, 61; harm reduction and, 79; intranasal spray, 47–52; kit, 46; method of action, 45; myths about, 63–66; obtaining, 60–61; response to, 55–56; risks of, 58; seizure and, 37; self-administration of, 61–62; storage of, 61; who carries, 45–47, 59–60; withdrawal and, 49–50, 56
naltrexone, 130–31, 134–35, 208
Narcan. *See* naloxone
needle exchange, 13, 61, 141–42, 145–46, 212
911, 53, 70–72
nitazines, 103–4
Nixon, Richard, 166–67, 213
nocebo effect, 108
novel synthetic opioids (NVOs), 103–4
NVOs. *See* novel synthetic opioids (NVOs)

occupation, as risk factor, 26
Odyssey, The (Homer), 114
opioids: defined, 208–9; method of action, 32–34; packaging of, 4, *33*, 38, *115*; paraphernalia with, 38; signs of use of, 35. *See also specific drugs*
opioid use disorder (OUD), 78, 121, 125, 132. *See also* addiction
opium, 114–15, 207–8
Opvee, 50
Oregon, 173–75
OUD. *See* opioid use disorder (OUD)
overdose: poisoning *vs.*, 94–95; polydrug use and, 26–27; prior, as risk factor, 29; recognizing, 32–41; responding to, 40–41; risk of, 17–30; routes of administration and, 38–39; signs of, 36–38. *See also* deaths, overdose
oxycodone, 7, 39, 98–99, 209
OxyContin, 87–88, 209

packaging, of opioids, 4, *33*, 38, *115*
pain: chronic, 21, 202–3; social, 156
peer support, 210
Percocet, 1, 22, 95, 98, 151
personality, as risk factor, 24
placebo effect, 108
poisoning, overdose *vs.*, 94–95
polydrug use, 26–27
Portugal, 173
potency, 8, 39, 90–93, 103, 169, 192, 202, 205, 209
prescription: for buprenorphine, 132–33; counterfeit, drugs, 21–22, 98–99, *99*; opioid, as risk factor, 20–21

prohibition, 95, 116, 133, 175, 206
pulmonary edema, 37, 58, 75, 140
pulse, 40–41, 54
pupils, pinpoint, 35
Purdue Pharma, 87, 209

race, opioid crisis and, 167–68, 210
Reagan, Ronald, 167
recovery navigators, 78
relapse, 125, 127, 210
risk, of overdose, 17–30
risk factors, for addiction, 20–26
Robinson v. California, 163
rock bottom, 154–55
routes of administration, 38–39
routes of exposure, 210–11

safe injection site, 53, 146–47, 175–76, 211
safe supply, 14, 94, 175, 177, 194, 171–72
San Francisco, California, 173
Saslow, Eli, 163–64
Schumer, Charles, 107
sedatives, 26
seizure, 37
shame, 77
Sinaloa cartel, 170–71
snorting, 39
social pain, 156
stigma, 7–8; addiction and, 150; conditions associated with, 152–53; death and, 136; defined, 152, 211; discrimination and, 155; fentanyl myths and, 109–10; harms of, 150–59; from health care providers, 77; media and, 157; medication-assisted treatment and, 109–10, 134; methadone and, 134; xylazine and, 107
stimulants, 27, 111–12. *See also* cocaine; methamphetamine
stimulation, in overdose response, 40, 48, 59
stupor, 35
Suboxone, 78, 131, 152, 211–12. *See also* buprenorphine
substance use disorder, 212. *See also* addiction
supply: safe, 14, 94, 175, 177, 194, 171–72; unsafe, 93, 175
syringe exchange, 13, 61, 141–42, 145–46, 212

Tennyson, Alfred Lord, 114
test strips, 95–96, *97*
thrill-seeking, 24
time of onset, 39
Today I Matter project, *18*, *164*, *192*
tolerance, 5, 28, 169, 212
tranq. *See* xylazine
transdermal, 38–39, 89
trauma, childhood, 10, 23
treatment, of addiction: behavioral therapy in, 130; detoxification in, 127–29; lack of, 125; medication-assisted treatment

in, 130–32, 147; methadone in, 19, 125–26; outpatient, 129; programs for, 129; residential, 129; what to look for in, 135–36
triggers, 121, 168, 212
twelve-step program, 13, 213

unconsciousness, 26, 36, 38, 40, 59

vegetative state, 80
violence, 65–66, 75
Volkow, Nora, 156
vomiting, 49

War on Drugs, 4, 14, 166–68, 193, 213
welfare checks, 29–30
West Virginia, 173
withdrawal: buprenorphine and, 78; defined, 213; from fentanyl, 91–92; naloxone and, 49–51, 56, 63, 65, 75–76; neurophysiology of, 119; stigma and, 77; from xylazine, 105

X-waiver, 132–33
xylazine, 57, 104–7, 157, 214

Explore Other Books from HOPKINS PRESS

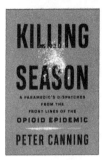

"From his ambulance, Canning gives names and faces to the invisible masses while reminding us we are only a prescription away ourselves. A must read."

—Van Asher,
Harm Reduction Coordinator, Cylar House, Housing Works

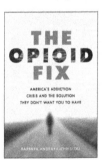

"This book is an excellent primer for anyone who wants to learn more about the history, effectiveness, and barriers to opioid agonist treatment in the United States."

—Anna Lembke, MD,
Stanford University School of Medicine

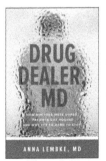

". . . a story with mythic resonance."

—*Times Higher Education*

JOHNS HOPKINS UNIVERSITY PRESS | PRESS.JHU.EDU